Love Me, Somebody

Love Me, Somebody

The Autobiography of

D. J. LeBeaux

VANTAGE PRESS
New York / Washington / Atlanta
Los Angeles / Chicago

FIRST EDITION

All rights reserved, including the right of
reproduction in whole or in part in any form.

Copyright © 1985 by D.J. LeBeaux

Published by Vantage Press, Inc.
516 West 34th Street, New York, New York 10001

Manufactured in the United States of America
ISBN: 0-533-06316-7

Library of Congress Catalog Card No.: 84-90293

In memory of the loving tenderness of my wife, Maria, who cared for me through many many years of ill health, crises, and tribulations. I offer my heartfelt appreciation for her noble understanding and for so willingly sharing so much of herself during the years of research, interviews, compiling, and documentation required for this publication to be finalized and this volume made available to you, the reader. Maria made sacrifices with devotion and an unlimited amount of energy, dedicating herself to the routine of housekeeping and her job, so that my work would go on.

Contents

Preface		ix
Acknowledgments		xi
I.	Introduction	1
II.	The LeBeaux Family	3
III.	The Day My Life Was Turned Upside Down	9
IV.	God Smiled on Me Once Again	23
V.	The Miracle That Wasn't	28
VI.	The Silence Came Early	33
VII.	And Then the Bubble Burst	36
VIII.	Into a World That's Not My Own	53
IX.	Into a World That's Not Our Own	96

Preface

For as long as recorded history, there have existed certain hatreds and prejudices born of fear and ignorance. This is not to say that these hatreds and prejudices do not still endure, but through the centuries, and because of the deep compassion, enlightenment, and love demonstrated by Jesus Christ in his ministry, a few of these fears have been reversed. Like all new ideas and concepts, the perfection of new thought processes is far from complete, and only more time and far greater enlightenment might possibly close the chapter of one of mankind's greatest fears—leprosy.

The earliest struggles to establish the first leprosariums (which were detention camps from whence there was no return and never future contact with the outside world) throughout the world seemed an exercise in futility. Gradually, through the devotion of dedicated priests and physicians, there came into being more humane places where the disease was treated and studied and every effort was made to find an eventual cure. As the twentieth century neared, profound changes had taken place and the cure seemed at hand.

It was not, however, until almost halfway through this century that medical science advanced to the point where there was hope for the victims of this disease.

The sufferers did not understand or appreciate all the work, research, desperate caring, and love. Not all of them survived, and of those who did, many came through their ordeal with such a shattered perspective that all life's experiences thereafter were viewed as personal attacks and persecutions directed solely at them on a continuing and unyielding basis.

For those with this point of view, not only was the meaning of life missed, but life itself could never possibly be appreciated.

Some were able to accept the bad hand fate had dealt them and go on; others totally ignored the years of caring and work for their anonymous selves done by people they would never know and refused to accept the fact that their very survival was a miracle and a commentary on devotion and perseverance by uncommonly dedicated people.

Perhaps one day a perfect holistic treatment will be possible for not only leprosy, but also for other more debilitating conditions that today offer little or no hope at all. In any case, this coin not only has two sides, but an edge. The edge is much broader than a razor's, and the dimensions are much greater. One needs only eyes to see.

Acknowledgments

My heartfelt appreciation goes to dear Marcy Scalf, who has been helping me with the typing and editing of paperwork since my college days and so often turned a sometimes kind of messy product into a professionally finished document. Thank you for sharing your patience and professionalism with a friend in need.

Special thanks also go to my brothers and sisters, who stuck by me through thick and then, even when their own careers (jobs and education) were in jeopardy.

Chapter I
Introduction

Acadia was the name applied by France to its Atlantic coast possessions in North America, which in the seventeenth century comprised the territory between the Atlantic Ocean and the lower river and the gulf of Saint Lawrence. The name is of Micmac origin and was first used in 1603 in a commission issued on the island to the Sueur de Mont by the French government. De Mont's colony was originally established near Saint Croix (near present-day Calais, Maine) in 1604, but was transformed to Port Royal (now Annopolis, Nova Scotia) in 1605. It was abandoned in 1607 by Jean deBiencourt dePoutrincourt, one of Mont's associates, when he was forced to return to France in search of financial assistance and, during his absence, the infant settlement was plundered and burned by the English adventurer Samuel Argall in 1613.

In 1621 Sir William Alexander was given a grant of Nova Scotia by James I of England. Encouraged by Sir David Kirke's capture of Quebec, Alexander besieged Capre Sable in 1629. Charles de la Tour refused to surrender, although summoned by Sir William in 1629, and was returned to France in 1632.

This kind of rankling and bickering between France and England continued until 1745, when the Acadians were expelled. They were given three choices: they could swear loyalty to the English, they could return to France, or they could take the arduous journey to the French territory south in Louisiana.

The figures say that of ten thousand who did not return to France, six thousand left for the South although two thousand returned. How many died on the trip south is not known, but it is known that many survived, continuing the same habits of living, save for exchanging the solitary life-style of fur trapping, in which occupation they had long been exploited, for a close-knit, clannish, agrarian life-style that became a more revered part of their pattern of living.

They became tenant farmers and share-croppers, who helped one another by exchanging personal crops and personal favors very much in the style of present-day co-ops.

The expulsion of the Acadians in 1775 has been defended as an act of military and political necessity, but it caused great hardship and suffering. The Acadians' plight was movingly described by Henry Wadsworth Longfellow in his celebrated poem, *Evangeline*. Historians say responsibility for the tragedy rests mainly with the French officials and the priests who convinced the people they still owed loyalty to the French.

As a matter of note, Evangeline Bellefontaine, who, during the rigors of the exodus, was unable to find her love, Gabriel Lajunesse, became a Sister of Mercy in Saint Martinville, Louisiana, only to have Gabriel die in her arms. They are buried side by side, united forever in death.

Chapter II
The LeBeaux Family

In one of those very old villages, a century and a half after the expulsion of the Acadians, the deeply rooted LeBeaux family lived much as their predecessors had. They had a small house and did a lot of "doubling up" for bed space, living interdependently with their neighbors, most of whom were close kin. In that beautiful part of the world, surrounded by the lush, pristine beauty of untouched nature, they thrived. Nearly everthing was a team effort, not only with the happy LeBeaux family, but with the entire small community as well.

Whether it was butchering, planting, harvesting, or building it mattered not. All these things were done cheerfully and as group efforts. If one family had plenty of milk, it would trade with another who had plenty of ham. Clothing also made the rounds, as did the good cheer and love. There was always singing and joking in the homes, and when the joint efforts were undertaken, there was more.

Fishing and hunting and trapping small animals for food was enjoyed and relished, especially by the young boys, who looked upon these activities not just as great fun but almost as rites of passage.

The conveniences enjoyed by people only a few miles from this little Eden were things unknown, therefore not missed by these industrious people. They had all they needed, neither their wants nor their needs were extravagant. Electricity, running water, and the like, though not unknown to these people were things they just didn't miss. They used coal-oil lamps, carried in fresh well water, and rode horseback or used horse and buggies for their transportation needs. These unpretentious people were more fortunate than most, however, their simple but comfortable life-style notwithstanding, for this was the height of the Great Depression and these families felt secure. They only lacked cash.

Though never having been exposed to museums or other sophisticated groupings of an artistic nature, creativity of the most extraordinary kind was manifested in the second son in the LeBeaux family, D.J. At a very tender age, I developed a love of nature and animals that was exciting and all-encompassing; moreover, I had an astonishing ability to discover accurately how things would work.

Sensing this, two of my favorite uncles, Uncle Yas and Uncle Oro, spent many many hours helping me develop these passions. I loved this and always knew that not only were my interests shared, but my love for these devoted uncles was reciprocated.

Uncle Oro taught me how to shape bits of wood, then put them together. After a time, more complex things were attempted, and one day, *Voila!* I had built a goat cart, and a good one. I used my two pet goats, Billy and Petite (after a bit of unwelcome training), to pull it. The cart was not just great fun. It was very useful for me, in doing many chores on the farm.

Uncle Yas picked up on the rare rapport I shared with animals. Uncle Yas owned and raced some very fine horses. With a true horseman's instinct, he knew that I had the potential to be an excellent jockey. The two of us worked long and hard training the mare La Belle ("The Pretty One"). Her well-conditioned body was long and firm, with a long, golden tail hanging just above the ground. She had blue-gray fur sprinkled with chocolate "jellybeans" all over her back. I was promised that I would be the main jockey. What an honor to someone so very young! The local horsemen were most reluctant to have their own animals race this beauty, because they knew they would not only lose to this champion but also to the ecstatic young jockey who rode her.

Joseph LeBeaux, my father, was a handsome, strong man whose strength and great energy, combined with deep love and affection, kept the family together. He worked hard without complaining and was particularly sensitive to his family's needs. It was he who taught me to hunt and fish for only those things that were needed for sustenance and to respect those that were not. My father was a quiet man who used a minimun of words for a maximum of meaning, and, for all the adoration I had for my beloved uncles, Joseph LeBeaux was my premier role model.

Mary LeBeaux was consumed by and dedicated to her family. To her, "The Family" was her reason for living and anything interrupting the continuity of her family or any of them ever being separated from her would be the ultimate hell. It was she who remembered the unspeakable history of Acadia and its consequences best, and combined with her own maternal instinct, this made her a formidable force, dispensing much love and not a few whacks on the rear with her faithful, omnipresent razor strop. To Mary, Justice was not only blind, but deaf and dumb, especially when she caught us boys smoking in the barn (a two-fold misdeed, as there was a great fire hazard in that practice). She also had the pragmatic quality for which the French have always been famous. She knew instinctively and never forgot the things that worked in keeping the family headed firmly in the right direction. She was a master at manipulation and cleverly used different tactics for each occasion as they were needed, especially where her sons were concerned. Many mothers would envy her success, particularly mothers of sons. Although usually used to control daughters for their entire lifetime, the old guilt trip was her most effective weapon where I was concerned. Guilt combined with copious tears was the ultimate in control for me, and compared with the razor strop, this did more to hurt me than all the fires in hell.

As with most boys my age, I expected life to go on as it had always done and loved every part of it. The only problem I have ever had was easily overcome and forgotten. When I started school, I had to learn to speak English. With the pragmatism I had inherited from Mom I took that in stride. After all, I wanted to learn and enjoy the wonderful things that boys did together. I loved school, and I loved playing marbles and baseball and horseplay and the like. From the first day of school, there was beautiful Gleanda.

My life was so full and happy that I always felt wondrously blessed. I eyed the future in the most optimistic way, with full confidence that all my hopes would be realized, but God had other plans. I sometimes wonder if he were as good a God as people said he was.

It happend late one afternoon. The family was together on the porch that warm April day. I was sitting in the front with my leg hanging over the side of the porch and right leg folded over. A sunbeam piercing through the scattered clouds above was focusing directly on the back of my right thigh as if saying "Look, I have something to show you."

A lump, quite visible, the size of a marble, with a brown ring around it, was immediately spotted by Mom's keen and watchful eye (trained by many years to catch any early sign of childhood diseases).

"How long have you had this? Did you know it was there? It feels hard. Does it hurt? And on and on she questioned me regarding this strange, unfamiliar-looking lesion.

I hadn't even known it was there, and once I knew, I just wouldn't bother about a little old bump. What possible harm could a small thing like that do to me?

To Mom and Dad, Mom in particular, it was another matter. They would send me out the next day to see the nearest doctor. Mom wanted this thing positively and definitely identified as soon as possible and treated at once.

The nearest doctor was in Kaplan, some seven miles out into the prairie and not too accessible to the community. It would take nearly the entire day in the buggy, so she prepared copious amounts of food—roast-beef sandwiches, milk, fresh well water, fruit, and some of the treats that were baked in large quantities for the home.

She was never one to go unprepared, and such a long period of time would most certainly necessitate sustenance along the way.

Early the following morning, Mom and I hitched up Old Blue and began our long journey to see the doctor.

It was a bumpy, bone-jarring trip along rough, sometimes almost nonexistent dirt roads that required nearly four hours of dust and discomfort. Had it not been for the melancholy purpose at hand, I felt this was something of an adventure. In my carefree manner of thinking, it was something I knew my friends would love hearing about, but because of Mom's serious and dramatic attitude, I kept these ideas to myself, being long conditioned to the nonverbal signals emitted not too subtly by her.

Arriving at the office of Dr. Latina, our longtime family physician, Mom tied the horse to what passed for a hitching post and in we went. We were spotted almost immediately by Dr. Latina, who sent us right in his office.

Dr. Latina was not only our family doctor, but a lifelong friend as well. He was about forty-five years old, dark, and rather portly. He had gentle hands and keen ears, which picked up various clues to his patients' state of health and mind, due to his great sensitivity. Because of this sensitivity he was able to understand and solve problems in general and those of his patients in particular.

The physical examination took the better part of an hour. It involved such questions as "Do you feel this?" while he was feeling carefully around my hands and feet. Finally, taking a book from his library, he read from it, then suggested that I go to the reception room for a while while he talked to Mom.

Poor Mom had remained totally silent during the examination. She had sat stoically watching and listening. Whether she had guessed the nature of direction of the symptoms or the tests, no one will ever know, but with her many years of caring for children and her intimate knowledge of folk medicine and many remedies, there was a good chance that she not only had guessed, but, with her practical nature, had most likely made long-range plans as to her future course of action.

After her private consultation with Dr. Latina, she emerged from his office. The good doctor had his strong arm around her shoulder in a most compassionate way. She was saddened and had a new expression about her that would become familiar to me.

Oh-oh, I probably need some surgery done and it's probably difficult and involved, I thought, as a child would, and instantly spun outrageous fantasies as to my condition, whatever it was, with the clues so easily read on Mom's face. At the same time, I couldn't imagine how surgery or anything else could be paid for on Dad's small salary, as money was one thing that was always in short supply. The doctor wished us well and bid us good-bye, suggesting we return in about a week, as he wished to obtain more information about the condition that held me in its mysterious grip.

Upon reflection on this early memory, I recall vividly Mom's dramatic exit from the doctor's office and the trip back home.

As we headed for the carriage, Mom walked briskly, head down, taking short steps, arms swinging like runaway pendulums. She was visibly shaken, nervous, and utterly overcome with grief. The message was unmistakably clear now. Something bad had happened.

The suspense was devastating to say the least. My anxiety level was at an all-time high, and I was almost wild with anticipation.

Mom was in a state of solemnity and did not want to talk at all. She wasn't the same familiar, talkative mom I used to know and was obviously deeply overcome by emotions.

With trembling hands, she quickly untied the horse, climbed inside the buggy, sat alongside me on the not-too-well-cushioned, narrow, black leather seat and pointed the horse toward home. It was trot-trot-trot all the way.

Finally, after working up the courage, I asked, "Mom, what's the problem? What did the doctor say? I need an operation—don't I?—and you'll have to take me to the hospital, huh?"

All question were in vain. Good old, usually talkative Mom, her gray-blue eyes swimming in tears, blond ponytail waving from side to side, was looking straight ahead with both hands firmly gripping the reins as if trying to slow down a runaway horse. This situation existed for a few more minutes; then suddenly, without a hint of what was to come, she looked up at the heavens and, with great sadness, divulged Dr. Latina's incredible diagnosis: "My son, the doctor said you have leprosy."

Well, I didn't know exactly what leprosy was, but obviously you couldn't get rid of it by surgery. Mom went on to explain that the doctor didn't know too much about it except that it cripples the hands and feet.

The first thought that come to mind was "Well, that's not so bad. I won't be able to play marbles [a game I loved dearly]." Then I thought of baseball and other games, and what of hunting and fishing? Well, after giving this thing more and more thought, nothing was all right anymore. It seems to me that I was headed for a lot of trouble.

Chapter III
The Day My Life Was Turned Upside Down

After a short silence, Mom continued her explanation of "the thing," as she referred to it, to a confused and more and more frightened kid.

"People believe that this thing is contagious. They will be scandalized by the mere mention of the word because of the ugly stigma, "unclean," associated with it, as quoted in the Holy Bible. They might even want to have you confined to a faraway hospital, a hospital especially for the accomodation of people with this thing."

My hands got cold. As a matter of fact, I was cold all over and was making a monumental effort to hold back the tears that were rapidly filling my eyes. Although I understood only a part of what Mom was saying, the tone of the conversation was terrifying and the prognosis, as she described it, was more frightening than I had ever imagined. Wave after wave of fear and panic went through me as the grueling description continued to unfold. The inner pain being kindled in my heart exceeded the worse physical suffering possible. It was also on this homeward journey that Mom began calling me "Poor D. J."

"What are we going to do, Mother?"

"We must keep it a secret," she whispered. "Don't never ever tell anyone."

Old Blue kept up an obligatto to this conversation with the clippity-clop of his hooves, seeming to be trying to get us home quickly. He had no notion of the turn of the conversation, nor did he sense the highly charged emotional atmosphere in the buggy behind him.

As is sometimes the case in shock, my mind was also aware of the horse and wondered what Old Blue could be feeling. I was thinking, *Probably his only problem now is to summon enough energy to get home and relax and to graze the range with his cow friends* [as he was the only horse on the farm]. *He probably will celebrate his freedom from pulling the bothersome buggy by taking a big drink from the spring.*

Mom snapped me back from this reverie by telling me that no one, but *no one*, under any circumstances must ever know.

"D.J., people would be horrified and filled with the fear that they or their children would be in danger of catching the affliction. But most important, the word *leprosy* terrifies people and will create an unqualified mood of confusion, and misapprehension among them."

The fact that this was serious business had already registered in my mind, and the ideas taking place in my mind and the admonition Mom had given me about any conversation on the matter not authorized by her were also registered and stored forever. It was a death sentence given out long before the meaning of life was ever learned.

How would I be able to hunt when a gun couldn't be handled with crippled hands? How could I put in shells, pull the trigger, and remove the shells? How about plucking and cleaning bagged game? How could I manage to do the things I so dearly love to do in the great game of hide-and-seek that hunting had come to mean to me? It didn't feel good.

What was the thing happening that could cause such hardships, setbacks, trials, and tribulations, not to mention disappointments and great physical suffering, and at the same time be invisible to all? The blows I kept feeling were all but unbearable. Yet the worst of all was the unmistakable guilt I felt. Even though there was no way in the world I could be held responsible for this new condition, with all its terrors, the guilt in my conscience was as painful as the rest of it. Many children, I suppose, feel guilt when stricken by an illness or an accident, but this guilt was magnified a thousand-fold within me.

In my great mental turmoil, my thoughts turned to my dear little friend Gleanda—Gleanda who was good and pretty, with a face like a doll and long, blond silken hair. It was she who had helped me learn to speak English when I started school and never made fun of the French-Cajun, which was the only one I knew and the one spoken exclusively at home then. She was an enormous help to me with reading, spelling, and arithmetic as well, This was the closest of friendships, and it continued throughout the fifth grade. We became closer with each passing year, and the affection I felt for her would continue growing throughout the rest of my life.

I wondered how she would feel when she first noticed my twisted fingers? Would she view me as a "cripple" and back away? I felt the fear of not being able to hold a pencil well enough to write "You are my valentine—D. J. LeBeaux" when we exchanged valentines, as we had each year since the beginning of school. And what of the other holidays and major events when greetings were exchanged?

In the meantime, Mom went back to her all-time favorite subject: God. "Have faith; God will cure you," she said, "Pray, ask him to help you. He's good; he will."

At this point in the one-way conversation, I thought, *If God wanted to cure me, he wouldn't have given this disease to me in the first place, and he sure wouldn't give it to me one day and take it away the next.*

Faith is one thing I had a lot of trouble finding at this juncture. My thoughts were taken up with worrying about coping with and hiding the problem from everybody. I didn't have to extrapolate a great deal to realize that friends, relatives, and the like would discern a change in my behavior before a change in my appearance and this would cause a great deal of curiosity. I well knew that I would have to make a herculean effort to act and react as normally as possible. I thought about things like the Tooth Fairy, Santa Claus, and the Easter bunny. When I was younger, I had believed in them with so much faith, only to discover they were pretty stories for children to help them behave well. I wondered and wondered about God and his plans for me.

Arriving home that balmy afternoon was like stepping into another dimension. The other children clamored around, expecting treats and souvenirs from the long trip that had just ended. Everyone was talking at once and asking questions that, in the light of the past several hours, seemed trivial to the travelers, but of great importance to the questioners.

Dad laid down his plow when he saw us coming and began taking long strides back to the house. He wanted to hear the results now!

The kids were disappointed. Too many problems had evolved from the trip. No one had thought of shopping for peppermint sticks, jelly beans, or little boxes of grated cocoanut. In fact, the provisions, so carefully packed for the trip, had also been forgotten, as appetites had been dramatically taken away and replaced by something that seemed to push the whole world aside with its urgency.

It was unsettling to me to see Dad put aside his plowing, which was so important this time of year, but I was so glad to see that beloved figure that represented such strength and comfort coming to me in my moment of need.

During the confusion someone asked, "What did the doctor say about D. J.?"

"Oh, not much," Mom intervened, immediately dispatching *all* the children, me included, to do their chores, of which there were many and for which there had been a brief respite that day. Mom whisked Dad inside the house for consultation.

Nobody except the participants knew exactly what was said in that discussion. Mom and Dad undoubtedly planned strategies between them stating the best way to handle those incredible findings. What it was that transpired was never exactly known to me, but it left an indelible stamp on poor Joseph LeBeaux.

When we gathered for dinner that evening, I saw a man I didn't know. The whole demeanor of my dad had changed completely. He was depressed, withdrawn, and seemed to have shrunk into another person. He sat at the head of the table, head down, avoiding everyone present.

I was beset with more guilty feelings. Jillions of thoughts raced through my mind. Knowing that there would never be any discussion on the matter made it that more difficult for me to accept. The inner turmoil I was experiencing didn't reflect on my face, fortunately, but I could only condemn myself and wonder why, when I was the cause of such enormous unhappiness for my parents, they didn't focus their attention and energies on the other five children and their needs instead of all on mine.

In that one day I had isolated myself completely from the mainstream of family living and social involvement, in a frantic effort to conceal my condition from the rest of the world. The persona was forgotten, and that was when a mechanical boy emerged.

My dreams and aspirations remained intact, but because of the new rules, the spark of life had changed. I would continue to go about my business in what I felt was the normal way, but my inability to verbalize these intense thoughts and feelings held me in tow.

We three brothers, Maloon, Darbee and I, hurriedly left the table that evening, not troubling to excuse ourselves, in order to complete our chores, but, more important, to engage in our rough and tumble games.

We played a game very important to us and participated every chance we had. We would throw a stick to one another and try to catch it in midair, sometimes risking a miss and a bump on the head. We would hurl it over the house sometimes, and the champion who managed to be the ten-catch winner was awarded with the coveted title of "Thrower." The thrower had it all: title, status, control. He was, moreover, the envy of all participants. We LeBeaux brothers vied vigorously for this rank.

Chores were a necessary prelude to the really important things in our lives. We were learning sound values through working, whether we knew it or not. On this still fateful day, however, I yearned more than ever before to be a winner of our game. My self-worth had been so diminished as to almost disappear completely, and I needed it to feel alive and useful.

On the way to finish our chores, Darbee and I discussed strategies for the forthcoming game. We had to go to the forest for firewood, and as we strolled we decided to sit and chat awhile. I casually mentioned to him that the doctor has told Mother that I wasn't too well and had to have a lot of rest. Then I went on to say that strenuous and exhausting activities should be curtailed to a minimum. I concluded the chitchat by saying, "Will you take over some of my chores for me?"

That was a mistake. He went into the darndest rage you ever

saw. He was furious! Darbee jumped to his feet, screaming and hollering bitterly. "You're full of shit if you think I'm going to do your chores for you. You're just too damned lazy to work. That's the problem with you. Maloon and I do all the work around here anyway!"

He went on ranting and raving at the top of his voice to report to Mom that I was trying to con him into doing all the chores. I don't know all of what he told Mom, but I'll bet he did not give my "honor" a vote of confidence. Going to Mother was like going to the Supreme Court—it meant the problem was of supreme importance.

That little guy Darbee was a tattletale anyway. He told on Maloon and I when we smoked cigarettes behind the barn one day, and the first thing we knew there was Mom greeting us with the razor strop. Pleas like "Mother, please don't" were of no avail. Rules were rules!

A lot of things happened that day. Some of them I knew about and some of them I guessed about, but more things happened that day, it seemed, than normally took place in a lifetime.

Bedtime was 7:30 P.M. Morning came early. In order to do necessary tasks, prepare for school, and walk a half-mile to the bus stop, six-thirty was the very latest any slugabed could remain in bed.

On the way to school the next morning, I could see the profound change that had taken place in my two little brothers. There was an unusually great pageant of sympathy shown by both. They were most solicitous and considerate.

Darbee didn't have a trace of the hostility he had so clearly demonstrated the day before. He made a great effort to show his concern and was awfully friendly.

"How are you, D.J.? Are you feeling well?" he asked. "Are you going to watch the little bunny rabbits, playing in the prairie, hopping around in circles, wiggling their noses, and standing up on their hind legs perking up their ears?"

Darbee knew how dearly I loved animals. He and Maloon would often race ahead in the mornings to the bus stop, and I would linger behind to observe the adorable little bunnies yearning to feel their white fluffy tails, which looked like powder puffs. I would often laugh to myself out loud at their early-morning antics. I envied their freedom from chores and homework and knew that their mothers were not behind them to enforce rules. Most important, they didn't have to worry about the school bully chasing them around to beat them up.

Mom obviously had had a talk with Maloon and Darbee. I did not know whatever she said to them, but did know that, in deference to her usual unquestionable authority, my brothers would comply.

Of course, I realize that they were demonstrating their love and compassion for me. I could clearly see that they were trying to show me that. But what I felt the most was a sense of greater isolation, an abnormal feeling. I felt I was no longer part of the group and perhaps was even doomed. The implication of "poor D. J." once again had surfaced. *What is going to happen to me?* I wondered. *Will I ever be able to love again?* I felt kind of dirty and untouchable. Perhaps I should be discarded somewhere and not belong to the family or have friends anymore. More feelings of isolation, reinforced by everything happening around me, took a deeper and stronger hold on me.

We boarded the bus, and after three miles of rockin' and rollin' over the roughest road surfaces in the world and another four miles of supposedly good gravel roads, we arrived at school. There was the usual pushing and shoving as the students scrambled out of the bus to play a while before the eight o'clock bell.

Most of the trip was spent in silence. I didn't push or shove or knock anybody's books to the ground. There didn't seemed to be any reason to. Playing games with the kids in school now seemed to be a thing of the past, and I felt that the good times I had had would have to remain only memories. Mother had warned me not to get tired or exhausted. It might make me sicker.

I took a hike around the school grounds. This way my first year as a fifth-grader in this big school in Kaplan, Louisiana. The Cassinade Parish School had only taught grades one through four, and I had had to move on. I listened to the happy noises of schoolyard play, a precious sound that would echo in my ears nostalgically the rest of my life.

I covertly observed the many activities as I moved around the schoolyard, because standing and watching would label me as hostile or some kind of "wierdo."

The familiar warning bell sounded, and the students rushed to form the mandatory lines prior to entering the classroom, constantly to the hand signals indicating the next step of the ritual, used by the teacher with great economy. This daily routine had become an important routine of my life and an expected one. There for a brief flicker of time I almost forgot my new burden as I went through maneuvers to which I had long been conditioned.

Gleanda was lovely as always, wearing that red-striped dress, with her beautiful long, blond, silky hair hanging over her shoulders. She has sat in the desk directly in front of me from the very first day of school till now. Each year the two of us, she in front and I behind her, were as much a fixture in the classroom as the blackboard. I was convinced that the good marks I received in school were a direct result of her devotion to me.

School that day wasn't the way it had been. What the teacher said in class sounded more like the drone of a bee than words. Occasionally a word or two came through, not nearly enough to make any sense to me. It was a one-way conversation. When Gleanda talked to me, I'd look into her eyes with the appearance of listening, but did not absorb much of what she was saying. Although it was not surprising that I should be so preoccupied, this further confirmed and reinforced my withdrawal and feelings of worthlessness. One thing was feeding on the other. As times went on, my marks at school floundered drastically, because of my inability to concentrate on my lessons, and this in turn made me feel stupid and inadequate. I ached to express my thoughts and fears, but this was impossible because of the code of silence so unrelentingly enforced upon me.

My relationship with friends suffered, too. I continued to withdraw from them and was unpleasant. I would ignore them when they tried to talk or engage me in their play et cetera. I had the response of a clam.

Gleanda tried desperately to be my friend, even after everyone else had failed, but I avoided this very special kind of involvement to the point of wishing that she did not exist. So great were my fears of being rejected once she knew of my affliction that I did the rejecting first, as I had done with everybody else. Down deep in my heart, though, I really didn't want to do that.

Minute by minute, I added brick after brick to the wall I was constructing to keep out the hurt and to hide the awful secret always within me.

The bus driver, Mr. Dover, that afternoon counted noses, and we were off to our homes. I thought this day would never end. I knew every one of the kid's homes, every curve in the road, every landmark, every road sign. The dust powdered our faces at each stop we made.

Mom was walking slowly to meet us. I thought she probably was curious about how things had gone in school and whether or not I would say anything about the way I felt. She probably also was wondering if maybe I had skipped classes. She didn't actually say anything, but was able, as always, to transmit so much of what she was not saying. She did, however, later confide to me that she hadn't known what I would do with myself after learning of my illness.

Her meeting the school bus was another change. She had never done this before. Every single thing in every way possible was changing and further added to jumble my thoughts. She acted normal showing great warmth toward me. I wanted to tell her that everything was all right, but she'd know I was lying.

That evening she prepared my favorite meal of fried corn mush, milk, cream, and coffee, and from that day on I was afforded the royal treatment. She demonstrated the utmost warmth and love, always with a big heart. She had great interest in me and was forever asking questions concerning my activities and feelings while admonishing me to pray hard, promising the Good Lord's protection, care, and love. She'd tell the other children to pray, too.

Each time something of this sort was said or mentioned I'd die a little. I simply didn't want to be special. For to me, my specialness meant having the worst disease in the world.

That evening, I took a walk to some of my favorite places, but somehow the charm had gone away. The red birds didn't seem so brilliantly red any more. The river had quieted down. The trees in the forest weren't murmuring sweet melodies anymore.

I was being caught up in a pathological state of mind. It was becoming so severe that eventual recovery from that alone was in question, my disease notwithstanding.

As I had been excused from all chores, I felt all the more useless. It was then that I realized that one doesn't miss something until it's gone. I had been doing chores around the farm since I was old enough to pick up a hoe. Farm work was an important part of my life. Now that was gone. I no longer envied the bunny rabbits' freedom, as I so often had.

My beloved dog, Rip, always at my heels, sat unnoticed. There was no pat on the head or scratch behind the ear that day. The poor animal, however, never gave up on me. I believe my devoted pet was not easily fooled and sensed his master's pains. He was always at my side. Rip was an excellent rabbit-hunting dog, as well, who moved only on command, though on this day no orders were forthcoming.

I had a number of fishing lines hanging in the tree to dry. I toyed briefly with the idea of wetting one, but soon abandoned it.

A new and more sinister thought found its way into my consciousness. I would do away with myself, commit suicide. I planned to get a tow sack, put heavy rocks in the bottom, along with myself, and jump into the river, the way some of the neighbors solved the problem of unwanted pets. My dying would hurt the family greatly for a while, but they would get over it after a short time.

After thinking further on the subject of suicide, I decided to keep my pocketknife in one hand and cut myself free if I got too scared and changed my mind when beginning to drown and the pain became too unbearable.

After giving it more thought, I thought, *What a dumb and poorly organized plan for self-destruction to end the problem!*

The thought of swallowing all that water and all of the attendant indignities associated with drowning became more and more repugnant. Imagine all those fish nosing up to the sack just waiting for it to pop open so they could have a free meal. That was just too much to contemplate.

For the first time in what seemed forever, I smiled. I laughed out loud at my grandiose plan with all its shortcomings and admitted to myself then and there that I could never in a hundred years kill myself. Fortunately, the thought never again crossed my mind.

Rip and I started back to the house. Dad was also headed in that direction, for it was twilight, the time of day when he stopped work and headed home for his evening meal. That's when everyone else made a beeline for the dinner table, and we were always on time. Dinner had always been a lively and animated affair, with jokes and laughter abounding. It was one of those things a large family shared, but that was not the case on this night. Excepting for the gurgling baby talk, a few da-das of the two-year-old twins, May and Jean, all was in pantomime.

The unsettling events of the past two days didn't interfere with my appetite. Mom's freshly baked bread was to my liking, and, as always, I could not get enough of it.

Bedtime had already come around. In our modest home, it had been necessary for us three boys to share a room while the twins and Joan, one of my younger sisters, were bedded down in the parlor for the night. Tonight Mom's three boys were three little angels. There was no more someone taking all the covers or someone getting pushed over the side of the bed, et cetera. There was none of the laughter, none of the teasing, none of the horseplay that usually accompanied the evening rituals. A truce had been declared. There was not a whisper or whimper from anyone.

The next morning I hopped out of bed full of animation, endowed with vigor, having temporarily forgotten the heavy load I had carried the past two days. It was not long, however, before I woke up, found out yesterday's problems were still here today, and began looking for answers that did not exist.

Days, weeks, and months passed, sometimes fast and sometimes slow, but always with a ring of certainty. The problem was with me. In the back of my mind was the insistent nagging about my health and my future. I had not yet experienced the many rigors I had been told of in connection with my dreaded disease, but my mind was really muddled and this was reflected most in my schoolwork. After being a top student with top grades, I was now the holder of the poorest grades in the class. I felt that this was because I was the worst student in the school and more reinforcement of my isolation. It felt so good when I could answer the teachers' questions correctly and when I did well on tests and reviews. Somewhere deep inside I knew that it could be done again if I really tried, but that would mean giving up my mental anguish long enough to study hard. How many people are there who have to hold on to an unreasonable premise in order to hold on at all? To me, having no guidance with this terror, the plummeting marks in school seemed to justify the great humiliation I was suffering. I was totally in the dark as to the underlying reasons for it. I wanted to tell them all what worried me, on the one hand, but dared not, on the other.

In the meantime, Mom began to tell me more and more about the disease, saying that it sometimes disfigures.

She described the development of swelling blemishes on the face and hands and feet and mentioned the short lifespans of most victims. She also mentioned that when the malady worsens, it stays with one until his or her energy, which is quite limited to begin with, is completely gone.

I surmised that Mom was getting this flow of information from the doctor. She stated further that she wanted to be fair with me and tell me all she could about the disease and its effects so that I could make the decision whether to go to the hospital or not. She continued by telling me that she just couldn't summon the courage to tell her own son to leave home for good and that that decision would be left up to me.

This responsibility was an incredible one for anybody, let alone a ten-year-old. I thought of hospitals as places one goes to die. I had already abandoned the idea of suicide, but any other decision making was not something I felt I was ready for at that time. With all my inner turmoil, it was all I could do just to make it from one day to the next. Besides, I liked living within the confines of a warm home and didn't want to leave. In addition to this, I also knew, or thought I knew, that my leaving home forever, for any reason, would surely kill Mom.

She cared for her family and children more than anything else in the whole world. The very thought that one of us might someday leave her was a source of constant worry to her. It was simply more comfortable for me to leave all the do's and don'ts to her as always, even if her decisions were not always tailored to my satisfaction.

The decision-making suggestion that Mother had presented to me did little to enhance my mental health. Already confused, I sank deeper into depression. The ever-present guilt was also magnified greatly. I felt this as a crushing blow and came to the adult conclusion that life was not fair, but I was in no mood to express this and Mom certainly was in no mood to hear how I felt. She was already highly emotional, but especially so when discussing the "bad disease" or "this thing." She had mentioned death to me, saying that I kind of was on "Death Row." None of this got high points with me. I felt that I had nothing to look forward to, but at the same time maybe death would be a way out. The only peace I had was when sleeping.

I didn't want to live, didn't want to die, didn't want to suffer, and didn't want to deal with the situation.

The routine of attending school and attempting to present a "normal" picture to the world continued. By now, I was using a crutch occasionally. I would sometimes make abortive attempts to participate in the sports and games played at school, but usually could be found sitting on the ground, pulling on my big toe—a habit I had had since infancy.

I wanted more and more to share and discuss my awful secret with someone, anyone, but had by now successfully closed out nearly the whole world.

Daily, careful examination of the spot on the back of my leg by Mother continued. During these examination, I was bombarded with instructions to pray.

I spent a lot of time looking in the mirror, scrutinizing my face, hands, and feet. My purpose was twofold: I wanted to well remember how I looked before disfiguration and was also looking for telltale signs of the approach of the disease. What I saw when I looked was a small boy with a mop of thick brown hair that was in need of cutting. I saw hands and feet that looked just fine except for a line of dirt under the fingernails that seemed to be always there. My habit of tugging my big toe increased as my thoughts, turning inward, were focused on the terrible consequences—not only to myself, but to my family as well—if the secret should ever come out.

It is reasonable to assume that my overnight transformation from a happy, carefree boy, a good student and a popular one, to a morose, brooding, taciturn person who radiated gloom and unhappiness had been noticed by even the most insensitive observers. Viewed through the eyes of an immature child, however, none of these things seemed apparent to me. I spent a lot of time believing that I was acting normally.

Time away from school wasn't too well organized, but it subtly fed my creative thinking. For hours I would watch cloud formations—mountain ranges, bowls of potato salad, and heads coming off horses sailing across the skies. There was excitement and drama in watching nature's storybook unfold its endless narrative, which I could have found in the pages of the most absorbing book. I was also completely free to interpret what I saw. Fortunately my interpretations were always of a positive and entertaining nature.

My relationship with Maskie, the family milk cow who faithfully and gently served us and provided for countless needs, deepened as I spent more time with her and the other animals, wild and domestic, which were to be found around the farm in super-abundance.

The trees and plants told their own stories and taught me lessons about things to come as they went through their annual cycles of turning green, blossoming, and shedding their leaves in the fall. I learned their lessons well.

Sometimes I'd find myself running wildly through the fields until I dropped. I did not know why, but I always felt better after this physical exertion, which gave vent to the extreme pressures that were forever building inside me.

During the times I was communing with nature, my introspection was of a positive nature that communicated itself to those at home. As my walks, runs and cloud watching increased, Mother's tears diminished in direct proportion. She smiled more and in general seemed to adopt a more positive attitude than she had previously displayed.

Chapter IV
God Smiled on Me Once Again

On the day I felt the heavens opened up and God smiled on me, I was fishing at my favorite spot, sitting on the riverbank, pole in hand, in total contentment. I unconsciously reached to the back of my leg, as I had done so many times before, to feel the bump. To my great surprise and amazement, I felt nothing. With feelings of elation combined with panic at not finding the offending bump, I searched almost hysterically, going to the sunniest spot on the bank and still found nothing.

My elation was as great as the despondence of the past several months. With a large whoop, I jumped up in the air. Rip awoke, leaped to the skies, and ran around in circles to see who was attacking us, and we both made a beeline toward the house. No obstacle in my path could deter me. Through mud puddles and everything else we went. Why go around them? It would only slow us down!

Running into the house, Rip and I were a sight to behold. Both of us were covered with mud and heaven knows what else, panting and gasping for breath. The dog barking and still running in circles, knocking things down, while I tried to gasp out the wonderful news.

Mom immediately removed the offending clothes and the offending dog from her house and took me outside under the bright sunlight to carefully inspect every square inch of my person. She searched diligently—poor Mom did—not only for the bump but for any other irregularities of the skin. After what seemed an endless scrutiny, my heart still pounding like a trip-hammer, I read the message on Mother's very expressive face. With a slap on the behind, she gave the go-play gesture and did her "happy walk" back to the house, murmuring, "I told you God would cure you."

I spent the rest of the day staying out of sight. Though this happiness was held close to my heart, I knew that once the news was divulged at the dinner table, my brothers would resent having my chores to do. Darbee had his own special way of letting me know when he didn't like something I did. When only a short time before I had thought that I had "missed" doing my chores, now it was a different story.

Nothing was said at the dinner table about the miracle, but everybody could clearly see that something of a positive nature had developed. Gone were the doleful expressions that seemed to have taken up permanent residence on our mom's face, and gone was the aged appearance that had been in our dad's bearing. Not surprisingly I was animated and had the good feeling of a reborn optimist. God was my friend now.

After dinner as the family sat on the front porch, relaxing and looking for signs of weather changes, I felt a stab of guilt of another kind. *Why*, I thought, *did I think God was my enemy all this time? He has given me back my life! Now I won't have to kneel to say my morning and evening prayers just to please Mother, but I'll really mean them.* With true repentance, I prayed silently, *God, I don't want to tell you what to do, but don't you think you punished me a little too severely with that awful news of my being sick and dying? You made Mom and me cry. It all seems so unfair.*

I was the happiest of the happiest and set out to regain those things that had been lost. I just had to do something about the terrible grades and try to reestablish the friendships so valued and that I felt I had permanently lost through my attitude of the last several months.

Dear little Gleanda, who had always been there to help and comfort me, was a wonderful coach and tutor. There were times when I felt that I could never catch up, but I tried all the harder. My teacher, Mrs. Broussard, was understanding and encouraging, praising my efforts and calling attention to the progress I made.

It wasn't long before the sports and games I had so enjoyed once again became an important part of my life.

Soon my contemporaries started calling me "Picket Fence,"

"Skinny D.," and other unprintables. I loved this part of my life. The world again was mine, and I was so very grateful for a second chance. I felt as if I had just been released from prison, and my whole life took on an air of buoyancy and happiness.

Even a hit on the head by the school bully, Harry, felt good and I accepted it. Even he didn't look so big and mean as he once had.

One of my favorite games was analogous to what had taken place with my new attitude. The boys simply called it "running." Everybody would start running as fast as possible and continue for as long as possible. The last one to quit was the "champion." In this race to "catch up" with what I had abandoned, the things standing in my way one by one fell by the wayside, leaving me the champion.

I wanted to be more useful at home, too, but that victory was a little more difficult. I would sometimes revert to the bad habit of sloth that I had had on some occasions before the awful trauma had entered my life. It became fairly easy for my brothers to lure me into a complicated plan to shirk such things as spending the entire day pulling nails out of boards so that they could be reused. Nobody favored that job.

Winter was approaching, good for preserving meat, and that meant that the beautiful hunting season was at hand. It meant that not only could I participate in one of my favorite activities, but there would be a lot more meat on the kitchen table, which was something to look forward to.

Hunting season meant also that the whole community would have one of their butchering get-togethers, where everyone shared in the work, the song, and the laughters. Old farm jokes they had been telling for years were told and retold on these gala events and were greeted by as much laughter and mirth as they had been on the first telling. Everything was used and at this time huge tubs of lye soap, the Mister Clean of yesteryear, was made by the tubful with the animals' entrails.

About this time a baby chick we had named Poulet started following me wherever I went. It had been separated from its mammy and found me fascinating. I liked to be liked, even by a chicken and cared for it tenderly. It often looked like a parade, with me leading the way and Rip and Poulet closely on my heels. A lot of good-natured kidding about me and Poulet ensued: "Big deal being loved by a chicken. You are ugly like one," "Bird brain," et cetera. Even when I went to fish, the chick followed me and found a treasure of good things to eat, insects crawling on the ground and in old logs. What a joy life was!

One morning Dad sent me out to hunt some rabbits for dinner that evening. It was cold. Clouds were hanging down low. This was ideal weather. Off I went, gun in hand, trailed by Rip and my chick, Poulet. Almost before I knew it, Rip spotted a cottontail, and before I could have the pleasure of shooting, he had caught the creature in midair, not permitting me the pleasure of getting off a shot. That seemed to be the beginning of a real hunt, and the prospects for the day looked quite good. It wasn't to be the case, however, because for the remainder of the day, not one more animal was bagged.

Finally I started home, feeling shamefaced for my meager offering. When I came to the barbed-wire fence, I dropped my catch to the ground so that I could lift the wire and climb through. When I reached out to grasp the wire, I found it impossible. My hand had swelled to twice its normal size, trying to close the fist was, awfully painful and there was a strange, unfamiliar sensation at the same time.

I wondered what in the world had happened to my hand. I couldn't recall hitting it on anything, and it hadn't bothered me until this minute. I thought it strange and thought I'd better get on home and show Mom. She had many remedies, and there was no use in this going untreated.

Through the fence I went. I walked faster and faster, little stabs of fear and panic jabbing me along the way. I remembered the good Dr. Latina's predictions. The hand quickly became more swollen, with indentations easily seen above the finger joints and knuckles and wherever I felt the pressure of closing it.

The moment I mentioned "swollen hand," Mother dropped the stirring spoon into the pot and, turning around, said in a loud voice, "You said, something about a swollen hand? Let me see. What did you do to it? Why is it so big?"

Her expressive face told me she was concerned. She had me

try to turn my hand this way and that and could see that there was no broken bones there.

After ordering a few more gymnastics for the hand, she told me, "I've seen this sort of things many times. You have caught cold in that hand. It was exposed to the cold weather all day on your hunting expedition, and having it hang down while you were carrying that rabbit caused it to swell. It'll go away, you'll see. Just forget about it."

Sure enough, she was right. After I'd had a good night's rest, the hand had returned to normal.

I suddenly realized that I had let my old fears come back to haunt me and was angry with myself. I was angry with Dr. Latina, too, for having frightened and worried me so. Hadn't this hand, after all, built a wagon and done all sorts of work around the farm and served me well all my life? What a silly waste of time to worry about it.

Putting my doubts behind me, I went on with my happy life, new adventure, discovering of one of nature's secrets every day. The sounds of the crickets, the frogs and the birds of the forest around me were nature's beautiful symphony to me. The colors of the flowers of the fields so generously used in the outdoors were a great work of art, a gift from nature's palette. This farm boy appreciated and loved these things.

Chapter V
The Miracle That Wasn't

On a chilly January night, the family was gathered around the cozy fire, flames dancing on the walls, there was no need for the kerosene lamps.

The early dark of winter made bedtime seem late, and together the family was warmly and comfortably sharing the final hours of the day. it was a quiet time, perfect for unwinding before it was time to retire.

The children were sprawled every which way. I was sitting in front of the fireplace, when I felt a bug light on my ear, I swatted at it, but nothing was there, nor did I detect anything flying away. My ear lobe smarted from the slap, but I was really more concerned about the imaginary insect that I had felt land on my ear. Had I gone bonkers or what? With the imminent arrival of bedtime, the incident was forgotten.

A few days later, my forehead began to itch. It felt like someone was pouring a handful of sand on it. After I rubbed it with my hand, the itching subsided, only to start again later.

After my experience with the swollen hand, I decided not to bother Mom with these new and strange symptoms. She, after all, had suffered so intensely when we received the awful diagnosis that I never wanted to see her in that state again. So great had been her suffering that I knew that whatever I had experienced was indeed pale by comparison. I only was slightly concerned that I was feeling sensations when there was none. I thought it a bit odd, but figured it wasn't too important and refused to worry about it. I felt a twinge, perhaps, but not genuine worry.

A few weeks later, however, while engaged in the rough and tumble play of a ball game at school, I was hit squarely on the same ear by a ball that had been thrown with considerable force by one of the older boys. So intense and surprising was the pain that I fell to the ground, screaming and writhing. Never before in my whole life had anything hurt so much. I wanted someone to make the pain stop, but it wouldn't, and when the agony stopped it was only for a brief time, I learned, and would return later, only worse that time.

I caught myself up short, realizing that big boys don't cry. I didn't want my friends to call me crybaby. Therefore, I would protect my painful ears and face from any oncoming missile, not allowing anything further to come in contact with these painful areas of my face and hands. Besides, if my friends realized I acted in such a dramatic fashion every time something was thrown at me, I would at once become the target of anything that could be hurled in my direction, and I wouldn't let that happen. I was beginning to take charge of my life.

Soon it didn't matter whether something took aim at my ear or not. It began to hurt of its own volition and was becoming rather red. My eyelids were becoming puffy, and when I examined my face in the mirror I detected that my cheeks didn't quite match. One was different, a bit rounder than the other. I wasn't entirely sure whether the difference was real or imaginary, but my gut feeling was that it was real.

In a few weeks the offending ear was unbelievably sensitive and the lobe quite red and thick. My cheeks were still swollen, and the edema in my eyelids would not go away. The face seemed like it was trying to reshape itself, and the ear looked as if it were "getting fat."

In spite of my nonchalant behavior, one day Mom noticed the brilliance of my ear lobe as well as its glossy appearance. She asked, "What's the matter with this ear? Why does it look so odd?"

I just shrugged my shoulders innocently, saying I didn't know. Mom didn't buy that and called Dad to come take a look at "this." He came over, viewed it, and walked away.

Everything in the room was suddenly very quiet. The expressions on the faces of Mom and Dad told me the whole story. I had seen these expressions before, during those first six months after my visit to Dr. Latina. The unspoken message filled the room and my mind, and again the turmoil from which I had just had a brief respite began to return. the weight of responsibility and decisions was again dropped on my fragile shoulders, to remain forever. The terrors of my condition had already been told and, although I had had months of seemingly good health, had never been forgotten. Back came all the horrors of isolation as though they had never gone away.

The damned secrecy was again upon me. The disfigurement was manisfesting itself with the changes on my ear, cheeks, and eyelids. The idea that I wouldn't be recognized even by my closest friends was becoming more and more obvious to me. The aches in my heart were started again and though, unfortunately, familiar, weren't any easier to bear.

The idea of going to the hospital at Carville was too painful even to think about. At home, I knew that I would be loved, if nothing else. It was exceedingly frightening to consider going to such a strange, faraway place where I didn't know anybody and nobody knew me. It was a condition that was all but impossible.

At that point I was convinced that it would destroy me entirely should I make such a move, so I decided that I would "weather out the raging storm at home and try to survive."

This time, at school, I did my best not to abandon my studies as I had previously done.

My "new look," that LeBeauxdachi look, was becoming impossible not to notice.

One eye had developed a marble-size lump on it, and I had the appearance of being "wide awake in one eye and half asleep in the other." One of my school friends asked me one day, "D. J. LeBeaux, why do you always wink at me when I'm talking to you?"

At this point, these symptoms had become an embarrassment to me rather than a cause for me to withdraw into myself, as I had done before.

Questions about my unspeakable secret continued. My peers at school wanted to know all the details of the rather obvious changes taking place in my appearance. They wanted to know whether or not my parents had consulted a doctor and all sorts of personal information that I still had such ambiguous feeling about. I was very unhappy about my looks. This time I chose not to withdraw, but to respond to all their queries the best I could, which often included lying. But what the heck?

I stood up to my interrogators usually taking place in the classroom prior to classes, with clever and almost plausible answers.

       Q. "What's wrong with your face?"
       A. "Poison ivy."
       Q. "Your eyelids?"
       A. "Rubbing my eyes to much."
       Q. "Your ears?"
       A. "From boxing."

Sometimes the teacher would walk in on these sessions and want to know what was going on. She had the same questions to ask, but didn't usually wait for an answer, instead going to her desk and going on with the business of conducting a class.

As time pressed inexorably on, even the brave resolve that I had espoused when I learned of the onslaught of my dread condition faltered. The strain of the recent turn of events was beginning to take its toll. My grades began to slip—imperceptibly at first and then somewhat more dramatically. My disappointment at losing the ground I had so conscientiously regained was another pain in itself, culminating in the ultimate humiliation of being left behind when the other students were doing so much better.

In the meantime, I became to think of my affliction as an entity with which I was at war. The only problem with the premise was that the disease was constantly changing its course. About the time I thought I had figured out what was happening, something new would occur, coming from the most unexpected direction and keeping me constantly off balance. I struggled, nevertheless, with these unexpected setbacks, valiantly and courageously. The great strength I had found from nowhere was awesome.

Unfortunately some of my dumb answers to dumb questions

backfired. They would occasionally prompt questions that otherwise would not have been asked. I had come to the point where I felt that the numerous questions asked of me and somewhat successfully fielded might conceivably send me in the direction I should follow.

I was wrong, of course, but was actively engaged in a game of Russian roulette with all the chambers loaded, even if I didn't know it. My distorted idea about the hospital in Carville didn't do me any justice. I was convinced by now that it was a real hellhole. I visualized inadequately everything there, from accommodations to the food, which I knew would be inferior.

In my mind I pictured the most impossible of prisons and activities that would challenge the Inquisition. Thus another argument for the necessity of knowledge was pressing. It would be much later before I learned the truth.

Chapter VI
The Silence Came Early

Mr. Doo was the man in charge of nearly everything that happened at school outside the classroom. He enforced the rules, dispensing justice whenever necessary. He kept an eye on the students and prevented boys and girls, smooching behind the bushes and disruptive kids' inflicting harm on themselves and others.

As I got off the bus one morning, Mr. Doo was coming in my direction, and, to my surprise, I was the object of his attention. Speaking gently, he took me aside and told me that the board of education wanted me to get the word to my parents that they were to take me to a doctor to find out what was the matter with my face He explained that what I had might be contagious not only to the students in class and on the bus, but to the entire school population.

I remember Mr. Doo's asking me about my face only a few days earlier, but I had answered him vaguely, giving out no real information, as I had been doing with everyone else. So accustomed I had become to these unwelcome queries that I had dismissed Mr. Doo's questions from my mind as being of no importance. Mr. Doo was kind, but firm, in his beliefs, and this time there would be no evasion.

The remainder of the day I spent trying to think just how this message could best be given to Mother. I dreaded a discussion of this subject with her more than anything else. I knew exactly what would happen when I told her and hoped against hope that I could find some suitable way to approach the subject. Mother would become hysterical and go into a long, tear-filled harangue, with prayers liberally thrown in, lasting a long time, and nothing would really be accomplished, except her causing a lot of grief for all concerned. But I had to tell her now, though the prospect was extremely unappealing.

All day I tried to put words together in such a way that I could say what had to be said and not ignite my mom's emotions too much. I was unsuccessful at first, but after a while I had a fairly good script in my mind and maybe it would work.

I decided to approach her as she was preparing supper that evening. She would be busy and wouldn't stop what she was doing to hold forth on her suffering at having a sick child. This seemed like a good idea at the time.

When I got home I waited for the appropriate time and went into the kitchen to deliver the message. Whenever I'd tentatively begin a conversation with her, she was far too busy to talk to me. Fixing supper for such a large family was a monumental undertaking, and, in her own way, she reminded me that, as the mother, this was one of her sacred duties, even though it entailed an enormous amount of work for her. Not that she minded, but it had to be done, never mind how tired she might be. It helped her to forget the many pressures plaguing her. This day she didn't want anyone underfoot and she didn't have time to talk.

It was rather a strange sense of relief mixed with dread that I felt at this time. I hadn't really wanted to give her the news, but cutting it off wasn't really the greatest idea in the world, either.

I'll tell her after dinner. Maybe I can catch her in a more relaxed mood, I thought, I continued to go over what I wanted to say in my mind, thinking of, them discarding one idea and then another. The next thing I knew it was time for bed and I hadn't said a word to my mom. So I decided to tell her in the morning.

I didn't tell her in the morning either. Now what would I do? Mr. Doo wanted some kind of an answer that day, and there wasn't one.

I spent the day at school trying to be invisible. I went to great pains to avoid Mr. Doo and, at the same time, resolved that this afternoon I would tell Mom, for sure.

When I came home, Mom was in a great mood. She was smiling and really looked happy. I thought how awful it would be to bring her down from such a happy mood with such unhappy news, but I had determined to tell her, no matter what.

I sat down at the table and began, "Mother, things didn't . . ."

Nothing more came out. My mouth went dry, and my heart felt like it was going to jump out. My hands trembled, my voice quaked, and my eyes filled with tears after those three words, and I was unable to utter another sound. Mom was extremely busy and didn't seemed to notice anything amiss but continued with what she had been doing.

I took a deep breath, realizing she hadn't heard my degenerative presentation, and decided to give it another try.

It didn't work. After a couple of minutes, I made a hasty retreat. Maybe tomorrow I could do it.

At school I was more determined than ever to stay out of Mr. Doo's sight. A good hiding place would be in the middle of a bunch of noisy kids, and I decided to give it a try. Another day was spent ducking and hiding. At the same time I was trying to work up the courage to tell Mom, and when the final bell rang I felt I had made it through one more day without a confrontation.

No matter how hard I tried, I could not work up the courage to tell Mother. I spent three days hiding from Mr. Doo.

Chapter VII
And Then the Bubble Burst

As I got off the bus that Friday, Mr. Doo, grim-faced, was there waiting for me. Mr. Doo was a good man and a compassionate one, but he had a job to do that was both delicate and difficult.

Taking me aside, he said, "D. J., you cannot come to school anymore. You are a sick boy. The illness you have is contagious. You are endangering the health of the children here. We need to take precautions to insure the health and safety of the students before they catch it. It may be too late already."

Evidently, the increasingly obvious and unmistakable symptoms I had exhibited during the past months had told the local people something. It is also reasonable to assume that these same symptoms, which I had tried so hard to explain away, had been recognized by somebody who knew what they meant. At that time (the early 1930's), when even less was known about the disease than today, in that backwoods community, with its complete lack of sophistication, fear borne out of ignorance was something that would give rise to hysterical mass fear.

I realized none of this, however, at the time. I had been caught up in the deceit I had been living with. To me, everything I valued was lost. I felt I had let Mom and Dad down and the fact that I could no longer attend school was the worse subdivision of the self. In my mind, there was no difference between being told I had to stop coming to school and being expelled for some major infraction of the rules. It was so confusing that every aspect of life was distorted, especially my thinking. This new wrinkle seemed ever worse. And what of my parents? I was sure that my own humiliation and heartbreak would pale by comparison to that which Mother would experience. Rooted to the spot where I stood, I was speechless. I felt as if I were dying and for something that I had no hope of ever controlling. I also knew that Mr. Doo knew, but couldn't imagine how he found out. The ultimate fear that gripped me was how, Good Lord, I was going to tell Mother. Such heartbreak was too much for my delicate ego. It was too much for me to grasp readily.

At home, I said nothing about my encounter with Mr. Doo or anything that had taken place. Nobody at home said anything upsetting to me either. In a way, this took off some of the pressures I had felt during the past week, but there was no discussion of me or my illness, which heretofore had been the focus of attention.

I knew I just had to tell Mom of this new twist of fate, but in the past although the week had finally passed and nothing had been said or revealed, I realized Mom would have to know. She was bound to notice when I didn't go with my brothers and sister to catch the bus.

All of us were up the next morning with time to spare. I walked with the school group to the porch and watched them go away without me. No one looked back. It was as if they knew we had taken our last walk together. I sat on the front steps for a while, expecting Mom to come out and inquire why I hadn't gone to school, but no such mother was forthcoming. *Curious*, I thought.

Hesitantly, I ventured into the living room, expecting all hell to break loose. I found Mom futilely trying to quiet down the angry babies, who were filling the air with screams. No sooner would she give one a pacifier, then it would be spat out, to the accompaniment of further yells. I didn't know why the baby girls were so torn, but the sounds they produced in concert were deafening. After a few more minutes of this spectacle, I turned and went back to the porch and sat on the rocker waiting for Mom to ask me why I hadn't gone to school. Any comment would be welcome. I simply couldn't understand why Mother was saying nothing to me and not making any reference to my being home or anything else. I couldn't believe that my mother, who so dramatized the least thing that happened, was so disinterested and completely unconcerned with my presence at home on a normal school day.

What had happened is that she had been told to consult a doctor about my swollen face and not to send me back to school until that was done.

I walked around the entire farm, looking at each beloved tree and blade of grass as if for the last time, because deep inside I felt that the time was drawing near when I would be seeing these things for the last time. I climbed the hill where Rip and I had spent so many carefree hours hunting or just running for the fun of it. Everything I saw recalled the wonderful times I had had growing up. Then I finally went back to the house. The others had returned from school, and Dad was back from working the fields. We shared our evening meal, and I retired early, as did the rest of the family.

I presumed that by now Mother had told Dad about the school situation. Not a soul uttered a word about my having missed classes, and it seemed that all had accepted the fact that my school days had come to an end.

It was very peculiar, and the weeks and months passed. Visitors would come and go in the LeBeaux household without ever bringing up the subject of contagious diseases or school or any of the grim things I had heard of. The secret that was held deep in the heart of the LeBeaux family seemed safe enough, and the fact that I was no longer attending school seemed to satisfy everybody but me. I felt a bit encouraged by this new turn of events, however, because I had really yearned to be accepted as I was with this new condition. Though this acceptance didn't occur at school, the community in which I lived seemed to be saying by their actions that they accepted me.

Then people started asking questions. They wanted to know why D. J. didn't attend school and were vocal in other areas as well. They disapproved of what they thought the family was doing. Many in the community had come to the conclusion that I was out of school because the family needed another hand to work the farm (quite customary in rural communities at that time). As I was such a small child, anyway, the people deemed me not ready for such farm responsibilities and were not the least bit hesitant in expressing their views.

The Sunday visits from friends and relatives became more distant. The relationships lacked their original qualities. The warmth had been taken out of them. The questions weren't answered to my friends and relatives' satisfaction, and the coolness became hostility. The LeBeaux family was regarded as having strayed from the code of problem sharing with their friends.

Then the bomb fell. The community learned I had leprosy! They stood back in horror. The citizens were terrified and let it be known that I wasn't wanted in the community. No one would come near me, and people went to great lengths to caution others to follow their example.

Standing a safe distance from the house one day, some people shouted, "Do something with D. J." among other things. Mom and Dad sent the other children out back to play so that they would not hear the things people were saying that Sunday afternoon. Dad became angrier and angrier with this new belligerence and made a few short trips to the front door to ask the crowd to leave, but change his mind. This continued until the man who for many years had been Dad's closest friend, Mr. Ale, shouted something to the effect that you could catch what I had just by sitting on the same chair that I had sat upon. Enraged by now, Dad went out and shouted back, "Yes, Ale, you son-of-a-bitch!" and returned inside without ever going back out.

A few minutes later, we looked outside. Mr. Ale was gone. Either Dad had scared him off or he had just given up—no one will ever know.

I looked up at Mom. Her lips were moving. She was silently praying, with tears flowing gently down her cheeks. Later she would alternately pray and talk. "When will this ever end? How are we to survive these hard times, being totally isolated from the community? Times are hard and we need their help."

The Sunday visits, a long tradition, came to a quick halt.

Mom and Dad did visit Uncle Yas, her brother, once or twice. My siblings, not being welcome elsewhere, played together the games they enjoyed and stayed out of everyone's way.

More pressing, however, was the fact that this had always been an interdependent community, each household providing the other with its special products. Now even this had been withdrawn from us, further isolating us, but this time in a way that jeopardized our very existence.

As sharecroppers, our lives were tenuous, at best. Now what

little support we had had from our contemporaries was being withdrawn entirely. Their love was missed more than all the vegetable, fruits, meats, and hand-me-downs that had been given us.

Dad really didn't care too much for the company of a great number of people, preferring groups of three or four at the most. It wasn't the lack of social intercourse that concerned him; it was more the disappointment in those whom he had long considered his closest friends and allies, both in good times and bad.

Mother, on the other hand, had enjoyed the company of a large number of people, which had afforded her the further opportunity to actively demonstrate her role as a most loving and caring person. This role was daily shown her family also, but she did relish the chance to display it elsewhere whenever possible. Certainly, at this point in her life, her pains were real, and being unable to reveal her agony to the world at large was a deep frustration to her.

Dad's strength was something to envy and emulate. He had the qualities that a young man growing up wanted to have. His physical strength as well as his great compassion and sensitivity were increasingly evident during this time of great stress. I looked to my dad for strength and guidance now and wondered and wondered what his former friend, Mr. Ale, had said about sending me to Carville. Carville, the hospital for the dying, for the unclean, for the rejected, seemed worse than hell could possibly be to the young me.

The neighbors made it quite plain that my parents were shirking their responsibility by not getting me out of their midst. They didn't want me there and went to great lengths to get the message to my parents about how they felt.

I, in my misery and guilt, didn't know which way to turn. It was not only me, now, but also the whole family suffering because of my affliction. It came to me one day that Uncle Yas was sure to welcome me. Hadn't he told me that I was to be his primary jockey? Hadn't Uncle Yas encouraged me and let me help train his beautiful mare, La Belle? Yes, I would visit him and he would help me, telling me how to train to race his horse.

I asked Dad if I could use the buggy and take a ride to the racetrack at my uncle's place one Sunday afternoon, a few weeks after the demonstration by the neighbors in front of our home.

Dad complied and I soon was on my way across rough, dusty roads to my beloved uncle's place.

I parked the buggy on a section of the road that abutted onto the racetrack, about fifty yards away from the finishing line of the straightaway track. I just sat there waiting to be noticed and get an invitation to visit my uncle and La Belle.

I knew that my uncle would be glad to see me, so I waited there as a sort of a surprise, so that when he'd recognized me it would be all the more fun. I had a few glimpses of him going about the routine of caring for his animals and the general activities involved with other horsemen before the big races.

Uncle Yas hadn't seen me yet. After all, I was a good quarter-mile away and not a very big object at that.

I saw him come out of the barn, then quickly go back inside as though he had forgotten something. Finally he emerged again, holding a long rope, which he looped repeatedly around the palm of his hand and his elbow. Perhaps some wild horse had broken loose inside the barn. When he had completed the countless loopings, he handed the rope to some invisible hand inside the barn. Then he appeared to start walking in my direction a couple of times, only to return to the barn. Finally, he seemed to be coming in my direction again.

With great anticipation of his greetings and invitation to come over, I began trembling. I could imagine the forthcoming conversation with his beloved friends and relatives. I felt the reassurance I needed was bound to come.

Now I stood on the buggy seat, looking at him at an angle. I kept him in my field of vision while trying to look unconcerned. I didn't want him to think I was begging to be noticed and invited to his home.

After several hours of this charade, I knew my trip had been in vain. I had given him every opportunity to recognize me and had extended the benefit of the doubt beyond what might be expected, yet I eventually knew that my uncle Yas, the one who had encouraged and guided me and loved me and given one aspect of my life a new and greater meaning, wouldn't see me anymore. He wouldn't encourage me again and wouldn't even acknowledge my presence after many hours of conscious waiting.

I knew then that my horseracing days were over, as was the intimate and satisfying relationship with my beloved uncle.

Reluctantly, I turned the buggy around and commanded Old Blue to head for home. I kept my uncle in my field of vision as long as possible, but tears and distance finally obscured him forever. I wept bitterly all the way home.

Arriving home, I dried my tears, not wanting to admit this recent rejection and hurt. I answered my dad's queries in a positive way and never admitted the disappointment I suffered that day.

Dad couldn't completely accept his young son's positive answers to his questions, but didn't want to cause more bruising of my already battered self-esteem by disputing what I had to say about this inimical day.

After this experience, I became really withdrawn and wanted very much to experience Uncle Oro's love. He was the wonderful man that had helped me build my little goat cart that I had enjoyed so much. But after this disastrous experience with Uncle Yas, I was reluctant to possibly relive the pains of rejection.

Three years passed. The days, weeks, and months all seemed alike. I went into despondency and never knew or cared about holidays, birthdays, or any other festive activities. The family, while commiserating with my frustration, humiliation, illness, and general depression, had suffered likewise. Food, clothing, and other necessities, previously in short supply, dwindled some more, Friendships of a lifetime disappeared like they had never been. Mom and Dad worked harder than ever, producing more and more crops and finding more ways to stretch the already strained family budget, not just for enough money, but for enough food to put on the table. As in all times of crisis, the family grew in strength and found more ways to be self-sufficient than anyone could previously have imagined.

I, in the meantime, sank to new depths of depression because I never forgot that I was the reason for all the troubles and problems.

I trailed my dad as he performed the chores on the farm and did what I could to help in caring for the animals, whom I cared so much about. Birds would come swooping down when they saw dad and his old mule and plow heading for the field. They had been conditioned to find good things to eat when Dad disturbed the insects in the cultivated soil. A mockingbird with a couple of tail feathers missing used to sit on the mule's rump or sometimes between its ears or on its back.

I was beginning to mature, and new feelings were beginning to stir in my young life. I was thirteen years old now. It had been three years since I had experienced formal education and the attendant fun and frustration. I had learned, a great deal since then, about how things worked on the farm and in nature.

New feelings emerged in my own life. Evidently, the disease had no effect on the inexorable progress of maturation; at least it seemed not to in my case.

The symptoms experienced had gradually become worse during the past three years. This was fortunate in a way, but unfortunate otherwise. Rather than the sudden onslaught of symptoms I had experienced earlier on my face, hands, and belly, my symptoms increased in severity, but did so much more slowly.

As the puberty period took possession of my ravaged body and mind, my thoughts turned to the one person who had meant so much to me for so long, the lovely Glenda.

She was magic, sweet, and good, and there never seemed to be enough adjectives to adequately describe her. Her loveliness and encouragement had been recognized by me as the epitome of all that was wonderful.

From the time I was six years old, I had adored her, and she had always, but always, been the one who would help lead or inspire the young me. Had she known how I felt about her, it would have brought a blush to her lovely cheeks.

These days, I thought of her day and night. The love I had felt for her before had intensified a thousandfold during the development of my young-adult sensuality.

Even though I had not seen her for three years, no part of my intense feelings had diminished. If anything, they had intensified.

I always remembered the graceful arch of her neck and almost wept thinking of the beauty of our past relationship. I could recall the lovely curve of her cheek, with her long eyelashes casting shadows under her deep-blue eyes. The sound of her voice as she had recited the day's lessons, flawlessly, would sound in my ears as though she were standing right beside me.

Gleanda was with me in a way I had never imagined possible. I would dream of that beautiful corn-silk hair tumbling over her dainty shoulders; in my dreams I could feel its delicate incandesence with my fingertips and smell the perfume that only she had.

Gleanda became my whole world as she had been before, only now with a new dimension.

In better days, I had elevated her to the rank of princess, placing her on my pedestal, as befitting her rank. If she had been a princess before, she was now a goddess. I traveled back in memory, reliving every moment that the two of us had shared.

I would smilingly recall the major event when she had bested all competition, becoming the "Queen Bee" of the hotly contested spelling bee. The contest had gone on for hours, but in her unflinching and well-bred way, she had remained perfectly composed, never displaying the slightest hesitation when it was her turn to spell. She had scored a major victory by spelling the difficult word *geographer,* which at that time I didn't even know the meaning of, much less the spelling. Although eliminated early in the contest, I loyally cheered Gleanda on to her eventual victory.

Always a gracious winner, she had been standing at the front of the class all that time, her dress looking as freshly ironed as if she had just put it on, defeating the previous winner, Susan, with great aplomb. Nevertheless, Gleanda had a kind word and a smile for her defeated opponent.

I was certain in my reflections on Gleanda that she had shared and reciprocated my intense feelings and love. Every word, gesture, or incident that I could remember was reviewed so I could find an interpretation that would suit my own feelings.

One such incident had happened because of a nervous habit I had, chewing on my pencils, leaving teeth marks all over it. Having observed this one day, Gleanda passed her own impeccably smooth pencil to me so that I could do the same to hers. I accommodated her wish and eagerly held it between my teeth like a little dog holding a bone in his mouth, imprinting the whole pencil and returning it to her. I never doubted that her giving me the pencil had meant my love was being returned.

She had shown her affections another time as well, when I was having a bit of difficulty turning the slippery pages in my book and needed a little moisture on my thumb. She had very generously put out her little tongue so it could be used for that purpose. It was soft and warm.

Another time I'm sure she wanted me to kiss her. She had placed her little hands on either side of my eye, looking closely at me, and said she thought she had seen something, a foreign object, in there. I hadn't felt anything in my eye that didn't belong there and had tried to inch away. She stood there a moment longer, her mouth about an inch away from mine, when I started to fidget, wiggle, and squirm and finally gave her a push away from me. I really didn't want to do that, but in my nervous confusion that's what I did. Now, looking back on the incident, I wish I could take it all back. Many times over, this episode was reenacted in my thoughts, each time with me realizing what a fool I had been in passing up this opportunity to kiss her.

These memory visits were not only with her, but with other friends as well. I would go over them until they had the quality of a well-used and well-loved book, pages floppy and creased with use, but familiar and comfortable and always a source of consolation to me.

Mom would worry about my lack of activity and contact with other boys my own age. In her own way, she tried to be helpful, making suggestions that I go hunting, fishing, or to meet Dad returning from the fields. She would offer to get me new fishhooks. Sometimes she would even accompany me to the woods in search of doves or other birds I could hunt, allowing me to go ahead, keeping a sharp ear for the sound of a gun and then hurrying up to go find the birds and pick and clean them.

The birds' destination, the stew pot, made my efforts a bit more rewarding, as I felt that I was making a contribution, of sorts, to the family.

Whenever she could, my mom would go with me while I fished, bringing along her sewing to work on. She would bring the babies, set them on a blanket, do patchwork, and alter and mend various pieces of the family's clothing on these expeditions, but she mainly went along to keep me company, hoping that I'd feel a little less lonely. She would fish with me sometimes, with a cautious eye always in the direction of the twins. Sometimes we'd take a picnic lunch and didn't really care if we caught any fish or not.

Upon returning from such an expedition one day, I was wandering around the yard, doing nothing and looking at nothing, when my eyes fell on the wagon that Uncle Oro and I had so carefully constructed. The little miniature of an actual wagon was setting forelornly near a tree and was almost overgrown with weeds. It kind of looked like a tomb in the middle of an abandoned graveyard. One wheel had rusted off, and the wood now had a weather-beaten look to it. There hadn't been room for the little goat-pulled wagon in the barn, and it might have been out in all sorts of weather for a long, long time. I just couldn't remember when I had last thought about it. It really made me feel bad to see my and my dear Uncle Oro's labor of love so badly neglected. The whole wagon-building period came back to me in a rush, and I could hear Uncle Oro's voice explaining how this fitted into that and why you did this to make that happen.

I vividly remembered how my uncle had told me the importance of keeping one's wagon in top condition. You must grease the wheels periodically with hog fat, and, if protected from the weather, the cart would last almost forever. What would the poor man do if he could see it now?

I kind of felt like the wagon myself, as if I had been abandoned and forgotten and nobody noticed or cared if the weeds grow over me, under me, or around me or if my wheels needed greasing.

That day, everywhere I looked I seemed to see that the signs of the more exciting activities I had enjoyed just a few years before were barely perceptible. Places where grass had been worn away by play were now grown over. The little belly-flip area (where I had raced, put my hands on top of the fence and landed on the other side belly up) for instance, was almost indiscernible, for the weeds.

My favorite tree limb, so fun to swing on, was gone, with only a scar on the trunk of the tree saying it had ever been there.

I sank deeper into the Slough of Despond. Everything visible reminded me of what I would never have or enjoy again. By now, I had become too weak to run and the use of the big 16-gauge shotgun was too painful for my now almost useless hands.

Mom came up with an idea and suggested that perhaps I might like to have a flower garden to combat boredom. "Near the house," she said. At first I felt it was not a good idea, but, on reconsidering, I wasn't so sure. It seemed to me that the amount of work needed for such an ambitious project was out of proportion to the end result.

Mary LeBeaux had been known to repeat herself on occasions, almost any occasion, and as she warmed to the idea of a lovely flower garden she tended to discuss the project quite frequently. What began as an almost offhand suggestion for something to hold my interest and occupy my time quickly escalated to a monumental subject that dominated everything under discussion and even found its way into fervent prayers. The more I resisted the idea, the greater the emphasis was placed upon it. Mom was not trying to be unkind or unreasonable; she just felt that she had had an inspired idea whose time had come. Mom felt that she had an idea to tell her son and, once she had explained all its good points, she would have completed an excellent project. I, however, wasn't buying. The impasse ended one day when I had a divine revelation.

It came to me like a bolt from the blue. If I went ahead and started to work on the cursed garden, then she would probably stop talking about it. With this unassailable logic, I solved the problem. I wished that all problems were that easy to solve.

I had long enjoyed the vegetable gardens, with their promise of good things to eat, and I had found pleasure in watching as the tiny shoots came through the ground and slowly turned into things that could be eaten now and canned for later.

I thought of how lovely flowers would look and, with my own thoughts, made the project acceptable.

To my great surprise and amazement, when the time came to start the garden, who but my mother did the clearing and the digging? That was the part of the garden I didn't care to do anyway.

It really didn't take her very long, and she broke up hard lumps of earth and refined the soil to accept the seeds.

When the seeds were planted and one by one they started to grow and produce the beautiful flowers promised on the package, I was pleased. This also caused me to reevaluate my thinking about resisting ideas. Not that I was to spend my life endorsing all of Mom's suggestions, but on this occasion she had come up with one of the best.

Mom and I were both very proud of and happy with the garden. It was fun to see those many violet pansies dancing in the breeze. There were two flower beds, running from the house to the gate on either side of the well-traveled path. There was plenty of fertilizer and plenty of moisture and plenty of attention paid to keep out weeds, and the results was a breathtaking symphony of color and forms that the more experienced gardener would envy.

As the inexorable progress of my disease continued, I gave more and more thought to Carville. For the most part, I was able to keep my symptoms from Mom, but by now, I knew in my heart that my disease wasn't going to disappear and that, eventually, I would have to go away.

My greatest fears centered around leaving the only world I knew for a faraway place. At the same time, confined as I was to the farm, I felt imprisoned by it. I loved the place and its natural beauty, but still the focus of my world had become so limited and my health so poor that the decision that had so unceremoniously been put on my small shoulders five years previously had to be faced and made.

I had already made the determination, even if I didn't know it at the time. It was the problem of telling my family, combined with fear of the unknown, that troubled me so badly.

For the past five years, I had relived the previous five over and over again in my mind. I could hardly recall anything that wasn't wonderful before that day when Mother and I had gone to see the doctor.

Not once since I stopped going to school had I left the farm, and not once did I talk to anyone outside of my immediate family. For a little time, Mom and I had been playing a little game with one another. I would make herculean efforts not to show the flulike pains and high fever I was suffering, and, with the same effort Mother would pretend not to notice. But I knew that she had and that she cried.

In many ways, I had come full circle. At this point I was very much the way I had been when I had first started school. Even with my cherished storybook memories of the way things used to be, I was really apart from them now. I had all but forgotten how to speak English. It was never spoken at home anymore.

Some of the neighbors would bring gifts of food to the family, tentatively inquiring about me from time to time, but the crisis that was upon us was going to have to be faced.

Mom had noticed new lesions that had appeared on my hands and elsewhere and that I had tried to conceal from her. She was also aware that I would often feign energy to do things in an effort to demonstrate a nonexistent stamina.

My face had swelled to almost twice its normal size by now and was purple. Whether it was a result of this or my confinement to the farm for five years, I exhibited rather strange behavior.

Whenever anyone not a family member approached the farm I would hide in a dark corner or run off and hide in the woods, spending hours there fingering little blades of grass, watching the fallen leaves rock to the ground, or tracing the path of some small insect.

I had a tree that I would hide behind to watch people as they approached the house. When they left I'd go back home.

Mother pretended not to notice any of this. She had grown during the past five years. She was still extremely demonstrative, but she had long ago stopped putting her own fears onto mine and a bond had developed between us, as often develops with people with long-term illnesses. It was strong and both of us took comfort from it.

Because I felt so bad and my mind was playing tricks on me sometimes, I decided, after not being able to sleep due to the discomfort of the disease, that I would just tell my parents I was going to Carville in a straightforward manner. Both parents were in the kitchen when I told them of my decision. Though not as smoothly as I had hoped I came out with it, only stammering a little.

My announcement was met with the obligatory hysterics, tears, and pleas to heaven just before Mom collapsed to the floor, unconscious. Dad had been unable to reach her in time, and she fell like a rock, hitting her head smartly.

Dad, the strength giver, with trembling hands assisted his wife to a chair when she had revived sufficiently and he had determined that no ill effects had been suffered in the fall. She sat there, sobbing softly as I went on to explain that I hoped the doctors at Carville might be able to help me get relief from some of the pains that were with me now all the time. I said further that I had spent the past five years at home and as that was all the time Dr. Latina had expected me to live, there had to be some help at Carville and I wasn't getting any better at home.

During the turmoil of Mom's condition and my recitation, Dad struggled to keep control of his own strong feelings. He was so surprised at the news.

Mom was still sure that God would take better care of me than the hospital and the doctors at Carville ever could. She verbalized every misgiving and nightmare she had ever had regarding this to me.

So piercing were her cries during this explanation of her worst fears that the other children, playing in the yard, as well as the nearest neighbors, some quarter of a mile distant, rushed to find out what in the world had happened. Upon their collective arrival, Mom hysterically told them of my decision to go to Carville, whereupon everybody began crying and wailing, holding each other in their arms as though they had been told that I had died, not that I had made the first mature decision of my life.

I felt as if I were at my own funeral, about to be lowered into the ground.

The neighbors stayed with Mom and Dad, comforting them, which they greatly appreciated.

I bundled up my guilt feelings, my swollen face, my painful body, and my isolation and went out to the woods so I wouldn't cause any more pain, suffering, or grief to my parents and watched the falling leaves tumble to the ground like wounded butterflies. I stayed there a long time.

Mr. Remo, Dad's employer and an all-around good person, had heard of my imminent departure and had offered his car to take me to the hospital. It was the only automobile in the community and was in good enough condition to make the three-hundred–mile trip. It was a nearly new 1936 Dodge.

On August 29, 1938, a dreary day, I had my bags packed and was ready to set out.

Nearly the entire community had gathered outside the house to see me off. They were silent and standing carefully so as not to touch anything. I had no idea how all these people knew I was leaving, but things have a way of getting around in a small place like this little community.

There were no good-byes to me or good wishes or any of that. The people just stood there as if they had grown out of the ground. I was touched by this demonstration of an interest that I'd never experienced and, with great courage, decided to reciprocate. Going up to a longtime neighbor, I extended my hand in a gesture of friendship, expecting a handshake in return. Imagine my surprise when the man jumped back as if he had been jabbed with a cattle prod. I was left quite alone, with my hand sticking out like a railway-crossing warning sign.

My already discolored face flushed deeper with humiliation, and looking wildly around, not knowing what to do, I burst into tears, sobbing convulsively. I further worried that Mom would feel even worse seeing me thus. I couldn't imagine how she would react when the "hearse" arrived to take me away.

I saw the car just before Mom spotted it. When she saw it, a cry went up that rivaled the heavens with noises. The other people, not knowing what was happening, were startled and, almost as one, dashed in her direction. Her wails and lamentations were so acute and agonizing that it was several minutes before the good people could ascertain the subject of such violent grief. The rest of the children, Jean, May, Joan, Maloon, and Darbee, were also on their feet, by now, adding to the confusion.

When the car arrived, it parked behind the line of carriages and horses the neighbors had used for transportation.

I hugged and kissed Mom, who had to be dragged, hysterical, from my arms. I shook hands with Dad, and my brothers and sisters.

Maloon and Darbee carried my bags to the car while I held fast to Dad's arm, as I was experiencing a sudden weakness and thought I would fall. With Dad's help, I made it to the car. Mom's firm embrace was finally terminated as I entered the car and the engine sprang to life. The whole family was in tears by now. And by now so was the large group who had come to witness my departure. The tears seemed to be the most contagious thing there. I could never understand how Mother found the strength to survive this incredible day's agony, which was surely the worst I had ever witnessed her suffering. God must have been looking after the dear woman, for how else could she have lived through it?

As the car slowly started away, Mom, who had her face buried in her handkerchief, looked up and began waving her handkerchief, then, with a sudden burst of energy, started running after the accelerating automobile, handkerchief billowing like a sail. The loose boards on the bridge clattered and I saw the last wave of the handkerchief disappear from view as the car took a long curve.

Chapter VIII
Into a World That's Not My Own

As we traveled the long road to Carville, I watched the familiar places go past the window, each with its own unique memory.

The driver was Mr. Trebuk, my cousin. He had brought his wife, Aunt Inema, Dad's sister, to share the return trip with him and, he hoped, to bring a bit of cheer to me along the way.

The prodigious efforts of my traveling companion to put a smile on my face were met with failure. The small jokes fell on deaf ears, and I responded to nothing. One part of my thinking realized that these were really good friends who were trying everything they could to make this trip pleasant for me, realizing full well what I must be feeling. The other part of me resented and blamed these people for all the hurt of the past five years I had suffered at the hands of these unfeeling people of the area. It was the latter view that prevailed during the journey.

About forty-five minutes into the trip, we went through the little town of Kaplan, where my school was located. Immediately my thoughts went to the years I had spent there. The students, the games, the teachers, and the fun raced through my mind like flash cards.

And I saw in my mind's eye the beautiful Gleanda. She would be fifteen now, my own age. How beautiful she must be now. She surely was bigger, but had to be prettier. I thought of her tiny hands, only half the size that mine had been. I could feel her nearness now. She would be sitting at her desk this very minute, 10:00 A.M. I wished I could stop the car, rush to her, and hold her in my arms forever. I was older now and felt I could probably find the courage that I had lacked as a ten-year-old. I wondered and hoped that at just that minute of intense thought, maybe Gleanda knew I was nearby and was thinking of her, loving her.

As we left Kaplan, I said a silent good-bye to the little girl who had won a place in my heart that was so special that it would remain hers forever.

I knew we would never be separated in my memories and in my dreams, but I also knew that, in this life, we would never meet again.

There was a lot of time to think and reflect on that long trip. My thoughts turned to Mom. I wondered if she would ever recover from the trauma of my departure. I feared that she might never again regain control of her emotions, after all that had happened that morning. My feelings were torn away momentarily from these poignant reflections by two things new to my experience. First, we were traveling on a concrete highway, the first I had ever seen, and the other was, we were coming to Baton Rouge, Louisiana. Never in my life had I seen such tall buildings, and I had had no idea there would be so many of them. I couldn't imagine such a place nor so many people and automobiles.

I also got to see my first train and had my first experience bouncing across the tracks as the car crossed them. The sounds were also alien—the traffic, train, people. What a din!

Stopping amid all the chaos, Mr. Trebuk asked directions as to how we could best reach our destination, then promptly got lost. After what seemed forever, we somehow got reunited with the Mississippi River Road heading south parallel to the convolutions of the mighty river. The road was old and in need of repair. Underbrush grew high on either side of it, often brushing the car as we passed through. In some places, it was so high it seemed to us that we were traveling in a tunnel. At last the weeds seemed to open up, like the Red Sea, and just ahead of us was a small sign that read: "Carville— 1 mile."

It was a tense moment for me. I was almost to the most dreaded place in the world. During the past five years, I had imagined how terrible this awful place would be, and for all my brave resolve and hopes of help, I inwardly was shrinking from the incredible nightmare just ahead.

As we continued our approach, about 200 yards to the right in the center of a large pasture was an enormous umbrella tree, incredibly beautiful. On the left was the levee. It was tall and wide and seemed to offer all the protection anyone could have if the Father of Waters became angry.

The levee formed a gigantic curve, seeming to envelop the large grove of trees and huge white buildings a short distance ahead of us. Vast, well-manicured lawns interspersed with beautiful gardens and grouping of trees came into view, followed by more and more of the same. Then groups of oak trees, encircled by what seemed to be comfortable white benches, provided a delight for my eye. The panorama was in perfect balance and gave the appearance that it had somehow all came together naturally.

Having expected to see the hospital, I wondered who the wealthy landowner might be and if he was in some way connected with the hospital.

The strains of the day's events before starting out and the long, uncomfortable trip had taken their toll on me, and although enraptured by the breathtaking beauty of what I was now seeing, I felt it was another cruel joke of which I was the butt. Why would all this be beyond my reach, like my friends had been and everything else beyond the confines of the farm?

As we followed the curved of the levee, about ten yards ahead we saw the large double wrought-iron gate. Across the top in big iron letters it said: "CARVILLE HOSPITAL."

We entered through the gate and parked the car. A guard from a nearby glass booth came out to greet us, and we informed him that I, D. J. LeBeaux, was a patient referred there by Dr. Latina.

My luggage was searched for the forbidden guns, whiskey, ammunitions, et cetera that were restricted in all federal institutions. The guard quipped that he too was a lover of fig preserves when he came across the jar Mom had sent with me. The bags were shut. I wasn't a wino, "gunno," or "ammunitiono."

The entrance to the hospital was just ahead. It was one of a cluster of buildings almost obscured from view by the surrounding evergreens that we had momentarily glimpsed from the road.

The receptionist directed us to the doctor's office. It was at the end of a long hall, and there were doors on each side along the way.

I tried to see inside the rooms as we passed, to see what they were like.

They were very small rooms with only a bed, nightstand, and chest in each. I worried that I would have to spend my life in the small confines of those small cells I saw.

There were people in some of the rooms, but I reasoned that they couldn't be patients because none of them looked the way I did. I feared that I might be in the wrong place, for this place did not seem like what I had heard of it.

My aunt and cousin were sobbing openly as they neared the doctor's office, almost but not quite echoing other performances back home. I knew that these tears and long faces meant that they loved me and cared for me, and the tears produced the usual guilt in me with Pavlovian predictability.

In the doctor's office, I sat as far as I could from the man. My recent habit of hiding from people had not left me. Given the lifestyle that I had experienced for the past five years, it wasn't too surprising that I was suspicious of strangers.

Dr. Yrean approached me, introduced himself, and told me that he would like to examine me. It was at this point that my relatives took their leave, satisfied that I was in good hands and in a safe place. I moaned inwardly, thinking of the long trip that lay ahead of them and mourning the fact that it was my fault that they had been so sorely inconvenienced.

Dr. Yrean quickly and expertly completed his examination, simultaneously asking questions after question (it seemed to me there were a million) about various aspects of my condition. I had no problems with the questions but was brought up short when I realized they were in English, which I still understood but hadn't spoken for years. I couldn't remember such simple words as *were* and said "teeeek" for *thick*. Words familiar to me wouldn't come out right, and when they did, my accent was so strong and my lips so out of practice that I had to repeat things over and over again, combining them with a lot of sign language, to which I finally resorted.

The doctor was very understanding and patient with me and spent all the time necessary to make sure that I completely understood the answers he was eliciting.

At the conclusion of these tests, Dr. Yrean escorted me to another waiting room, telling me to be seated and that someone would be in shortly to talk to me.

The doctor was as good as his word. I had seen a lot of peculiar things during my life on earth, but here at Carville the things I had observed during the short period of time I had been there were things for which I had been totally unprepared.

The presence who entered the room was like nothing I had ever imagined. I didn't know exactly, but I thought it was a she. Nothing was visible except for face and hands, which were scrubbed clean. There was a headdress (I assumed it was a headdress and not part of the head itself), which looked for all the world like a great big butterfly flexing its long white wings prior to takeoff. The garment this being wore, which extended form chin to foot in great, billowing pleats, was dark-blue. The sleeves went clear to the hands.

The voice was kind and well modulated, and it was then that I realized that my guess of the gender of this being had been correct. It was a she. She was a Roman Catholic nun. I, unlike many other people, would, for as long as I would live, never, ever forget the first time I laid eyes on a nun. It was an experience unlike any I had ever had and unlike any I would ever have. She was mind-boggling and awesome, and it was probably a good thing for me that my English was so restrained and I was dumbstruck.

When the nun introduced herself to me, I remembered to close my mouth. I had no idea how long it had been gaping open, and in my efforts to compose myself after this unexpected experience, I forgot, for once, to be embarrassed and feel guilty. The shock treatment I had just had eased me into the interviews to follow as nothing else could have done. In my amazement, I answered questions without hesitation and made sense most of the time.

She introduced herself as Sister Agnes. I knew I didn't have any sisters there; they were back home on the farm.

When she asked me my name, I was surprised I remembered it, but I did and said, "D. J. LeBeaux, ma'am."

She was a member of the Order of Saint Vincent De Paul, an order that had dedicated itself to the care of the patients at Carville. Sister Agnes went on to ask the usual questions one is asked on entering any hospital. They weren't particularly interesting to me, but when the queries stopped and she began telling me about the nature of my accommodations and the living arrangements, my ears perked up and she had my full attention. But this time it wasn't because of her unfamiliar attire.

She proceeded to tell me about the "Kids' House," where I would be living with boys my own age. She mentioned also the activities they had for the residents, which I would be sharing with my new friends. There were movies (which I had never before seen), tennis, golf, and bicycling, and the list went on and on.

"Pop Smith" was in charge of the Kids' House, and he was the one who made sure things went as they should.

I learned about the four boys I would be living with. They were Adam, Racso, Henry, and little Werdna. Sister Agnes warned me about a couple of the big boys who were a disciplinary problem. They didn't always respect the rules there, and she suggested to me that I avoid doing those things that they did so that I wouldn't get into the same situation they were in, whatever that was.

I learned that my medication would be a drug called Chalmoogra Oil and it would be in capsule form and taken with each meal and at bedtime. The medication would be given out by Sister Carmen, who would see to it that everyone received the correct dosage.

For the very first time, I heard something positive about my disease and about myself. There was help available, and there was no need to worry about breaking people's hearts or causing them needless agony or hiding or lying or any of those things I had been doing for such a long time.

The people here weren't cruel or cold, and the things I was discovering from the very first day here were unbelievable. The best I had ever hoped for was that one day I would be gone, as though my life had never happened. Now here I was, talking to this strange angel in her unusual attire, and a whole new world was opening up to me. This Sister Agnes certainly had done something for my life besides scaring me half to death.

That night, I was to sleep in the infirmary since it was too late to go to the dorm where I was to live for a while. I couldn't believe the things that had happened that day. The new and incredible experiences I had had were almost impossible to assimilate in such a short period.

Sister Agnes had promised me that the next morning I would be personally conducted around the entire place and shown every facility from living quarters to the areas set aside for recreation. Not having freed myself from the long-established and convoluted guilt, I eschewed the realization that the horror stories I had heard about this place were false. The people who had told me this had possibly, been motivated by love, but affected by fear or ignorance, but whatever the reason, I had been crippled by this mendacity and suffered from it far more than from my disease.

For the first time in my life, I slept in a bed not my own, in a place not my home.

After breakfast the next morning, I met Henry, a boy about my own age. He was to conduct the tour and explain the rules to me.

The interiors of the buildings were as attractive as the exteriors. The place was enormous, and not only did I see rooms and buildings the likes of which I had never imagined, but these places had names I had to try to remember. I had never ever heard of golf or tennis or volleyball, and though I was intrigued by and enthusiastic about learning some of these wonderous new activities, my head felt like it was filled with a swarm of bees, as all the new things and places and names for them tried to find a place in my conscious memory. At the same time my new friend was giving his narrative, I was struggling with the unfamiliar language, doing a seesaw of English-French, French-English in my head. I hoped that the eventual accommodation of English in my thinking and speaking wouldn't take too long.

Other data were assailing me about which many of the other residents had never had a second thought. I had to learn how to operate such complicated things as light switches and water faucets. As I was totally unfamiliar with electrically operated lights, lamps, and the like, handling their controls was very difficult. I could never seem to remember which way off and which way on or which handle was hot or which was cold. The flush toilet provided me with no end of fascination, as did the shower, which frightened me the first time it was turned on.

The rules seemed endless. Although they were for the benefit of the patients there, I had the uncomfortable feeling that the violations of these restrictions would be followed by consequences as new and unimagined as this place was to me. *Whatever punishment meted out by this overwhelming place must be direct indeed,* I thought.

The recitation of rules was interrupted by our arrival at the "Kids' House." It was well kept and neat, and its number was 14. My new friend showed me to my room (imagine, my own room!). It was a very nice room. I even had my own personal lavatory, with its confusing handles. I had never ever seen inlaid linoleum before and couldn't imagine how they got the floor to look so shiny and bright. At first I didn't feel right walking on it. The painted walls looked so nice, and there was my neatly made bed waiting with a nightstand and my very own chest of drawers, where I could put the things that didn't go in the closet, beside it. Imagine my surprise upon finding that everything had already been put away for me.

I wondered if I was going to have as much trouble going to sleep each night as I had the previous night. Sleeping alone was a new experience for me, and I thought of my brothers.

Continuing the tour, I was introduced to Pop Smith, head honcho and all-around important person. All the boys stood in awe of Pop Smith. He knew important people, and because of his exalted position, rumors abounded of his prowess and great knowledge of just about everything.

Rasco was introduced to me as we were walking along a long corridor. Rasco had the proud distinction of owning a BB gun. He'd lend the gun to friends who were nice to him, provided that the borrowers supplied their own ammunition. It was obviously important that Rasco's friendship be carefully cultivated and maintained. This young man enjoyed a unique and enviable position.

There was another "dignitary" as well occupying a top position in the organization. His name was Adam Ognimo. Although the same age as me, Adam was an oldtimer at Carville, having come there at the age of ten. He was a known intellectual and excellent mover.

Because of his demonstrated leadership abilities, he had been selected to serve as group leader. He enforced the 10:00 P.M. curfew with nightly bed checks and make sure that everybody was up in the morning and kept their own rooms in order. He oversaw the making out of laundry lists and doing the laundry and made sure that we all attended church services on Sundays and special holidays.

To my surprise and relief, I discovered that all the boys were Catholic, so we all would attend services in a group.

As we boys became a little more comfortable with one another, we volunteered various tidbits of personal history, comparing notes about family and home. Although we would jokingly refer to the amount of time different people had lived at Carville, we carefully avoided any mention of when anyone would be leaving or in what manner. There was some shared wisdom among us as to the advisability of never missing mass on any Holy Day of Obligation. The nurses at Carville consisted entirely of Sisters of Saint Vincent de Paul and were not at all sympathetic or understanding about a Catholic missing or arriving late to mass. Although their vows included caring for the sick, as they were doing, the vows didn't include any show of mercy to a baptized Catholic who did not enthusiastically practice his religion. It was said that if even a minor infraction took place, they would come swooping down on you like huge, blue birds, and God alone knew what would happen in addition to the rule breaker's receiving a vigorous admonition. Other inside information from the boys included the fact that if anyone had been baptized a Catholic and didn't like to go to mass, the sisters would surely find out about it and fearlessly enforce church attendance. The boys seemed to feel that this was some divinely inspired gift that the nuns had. In all probability, they merely looked at the admission records, giving special attention to the Catholics. The Protestants had their own ways of enforcing things.

I took all this in and vowed to myself that I would never do anything to incur the wrath of the sisters, particularly at the very beginning of my stay. I wanted to do anything and everything to recover from my illness and return to the bosom of my family.

In the midst of the series of things going on, Rasco gave a shout, jumping straight up. I thought *My God! He must be in awful pain*. He really wasn't; he had just had an idea and this was his way of letting us all know. He thought that we could all take the bicycles, with someone carrying me on his handlebars, and give me a more detailed view of the place. The suggestion was enthusiastically received by all, and out we rushed to the suggested means of transportation.

Hopping on the two-wheelers, we set out in the general direction of the main gate, through which I had entered the day before.

As we cruised along awhile, a beautiful brick church came unto view. It was the Catholic church. All around it was the most beautiful garden I had ever seen. It reminded me of the one that Mom and I had planted back home, except that this one was much larger and better cared for. I recognized some of the flowers, but not all of them. The riot of color was exquisitely moving.

The roses, and all of the other flowers as well were pruned and kept in perfect blooming condition. I couldn't believe it when, on looking at the earth from which these lovely flowers were growing, I saw that there was not a leaf, twig, pebble, or even bugs. The work that maintained such perfection deemed to me beyond mortal flesh. Of course, I didn't know it at the time that the intrusion of anything unwelcome in the garden seldom happened when the nuns were in charge of it.

We made a careful inspection of the place, inside and out, each new sight rivaling the last in its beauty. I loved it and wanted to stay and just drink it all in, but the boys had more to show me, so, vowing to return alone when I could stay longer, I went with them. Just across the entranceway from the Catholic church stood the Protestant chapel. It was a lovely white masonry building shaded by tall trees all around. It too was decorative, with walks that led directly to the front of the church.

Inspecting the outside of the church, I found it to be pretty and inspiring. It, like the one I had just left, seemed to be holding out its arms, just waiting for worshippers to enter.

One word kept repeating itself to me every time I saw anything at this place, and it was always the first to come to mind: *clean*. Every single thing, from the lawns to the buildings, was so clean. The care of everything at Carville was painstakingly meticulous. I didn't realize at the time that the grass and other plants on the lawns there also served the purpose of keeping down the dust and discouraging weeds. The humidity helped in that it had the added benefit of encouraging plant growth.

I wondered why any of the residents there would avoid church services when they were held in such beautiful places as I was seeing. Just being in the buildings gave me a sense of peace and tranquility. That alone was nearly enough to restore my soul and bring me contentment. Now the thought of God would never be the same. The idea of a creator who could allow this beauty to occur was elevated to quite another level than that I had felt previously.

We went on to the canteen, where all purchases at Carville were made. The power plant came next. That was where the mysterious electricity I was learning about was manufactured. As my friends explained all this to me, I marveled at the immensity of it all.

The boys took me around to about thirty houses, all connected by screened-in, covered walkways like the ones we had traveled on to see the churches. I couldn't imagine that there could be more to see.

This area of the compound was called the "Front" because it was where most of the activities were centered.

Leaving the Front and the smooth, enclosed walkways we had been traveling on, we began traveling on a more hazardous dirt road, which led to the area referred to as the "Back" was altogether rural, and I thought of the farm.

Located in the Back was a large dairy farm where I saw a herd of healthy, well-fed Holsteins. Their lowing was music to my ears. Even the cow manure that smelled so offensive to the boys smelled good to me.

To the right of the dairy were acres and acres of vegetable fields. As there had been a harvest recently, there wasn't a great deal to see, but there was the promise of good meals to come.

Farther on there was a giant poultry farm. I saw a big iron pot used to boil water for cleaning the birds and otherwise preparing them for consumption by the Carville population.

I was delighted by all of this. Loving farm life as I did, this was wonderful. I had thought I'd never be on a farm again, and now I was in the middle of the farm of all farms.

This still wasn't all there was to see. Behind all of this was even more. It was accessible only by crawling through a big barbed-wire fence. There were dense undergrowth and an almost impenetrable forest. There resided the denizens of the swamps. This was a place both exciting and frightening, and we loved it. This was a wild and savage area, full of adventures, at least in the imagination.

For a while, I stood there drinking it all in. Finally, we got back on our bikes and pedaled back to our quarters.

Upon arriving at our starting point, everyone went his own way. I was glad because I wanted to spend some time alone in my new room learning things.

So much had happened to me that day. Earlier in the day when we had first started on the rounds, I had been given information I thought I would never learn and had been shown a life I had never imagined. Now, after this latest tour, a mixture of delight was experienced, mixed with something else.

It was incredible that these boys who were my own age should understand and accept so many things that were totally unfamiliar and incomprehensible to me. I wondered if they thought me ignorant and if they would withhold their friendship for that reason.

Reflecting on the afternoon's activities made me uncomfortable. I had overheard comments in which I had been described as a "buggy boy" and "chicken lover." I saw from the corner of my eyes a few faces smirking because of my strong French accent. I wanted to be back with my family on the farm and already knew that I wouldn't fit into this new place in spite of the new and exciting things I had seen that day. Because of all the excitement about the farms I had seen earlier in the Back, the other boys thought I was crazy. They didn't have the slightest interest in the things that I had found so marvelous and exciting.

Had I not spent such a long time being in both physical and mental isolation, I might have been able to handle this, but the fact was that I had been isolated and now when I had a chance to lead a life with far more freedom to learn and explore new things and experiences, I had begun by getting back into the old mental pattern with which I was so comfortable by now. My insecurities were so great that had I not overheard comments that I immediately interpreted as unfriendly, hostile, and threatening, I most certainly would have found something else to apply the same meaning to. My retreat from people was so ingrained by now that the prospect of recuperating from what was considered an incurable, fatal illness seemed much greater than the possibility of recovery from the state of deep unhappiness and suspicion.

In the privacy of my room, after making sure that nobody was around, I rehearsed the use of the light switches. At first when I tried using them, I thought something would happen to me and was so tentative in pressing them that they wouldn't go to the positions to turn off and on. Finally, after many tries, things began to work. There was an electric fan in my room that seemed more dangerous, but after many tries it too began to perform. I kept experimenting with the other things and finally mastered their use. I was scared to death that I was going to break or ruin some of these things, but took the risk rather than risk laughter at my expense if I wasn't able to do them correctly.

At the dining hall that evening, I was to encounter still another new situation. The meals there were served buffet style. There were many, many dishes with which I was unfamiliar, having no idea what they were or what they tasted like. I thought if I took something I didn't like or couldn't eat, I might be the subject of further derision, so I took a few slices of bread and some milk for my meal.

At home, I liked to crumble the bread in a bowl and pour milk over it, but I had that uneasy feeling about this place that people would make fun of me and laugh at me if I did that. So I just ate the bread whole.

With that nourishment under my belt, I prepared for bed. I couldn't get the shower to work, so I used the basin in my room for a sponge bath. I said the usual prayers before getting into bed and prayed to God for a few minutes of peace, for the disease to leave me, and for me to go home soon and forever.

The next morning I decided to go over to the canteen, which was next to the post office and a favorite gathering place for the people awaiting their mail. There was a lot of laughter and kidding going on there most of the time, but especially just before the mail arrived.

I was obsessed with trying to found out what the approximate stay at Carville was and what sort of outlook for eventual recovery there was. Again, I heard the bantering about the two, five, ten, or fifteen years that some of the people had been confined.

Only about a week before, I had been telling my parents that I had already lived longer than the doctor had predicted, but I wasn't thinking about that just now. I had only been at Carville less than a day and already was not only failing to remember the reason I had come, but had returned to my customary attitude.

While I was in the canteen, an elderly man engaged me in conversation, and I felt certain to get some information during our talk. Mr. Sellew was not to say the things I wanted to hear, however. He went to great pains to let me know that the prospects of leaving were practically nil. Oh yes, there had been some who had gone AWOL from time to time, but they had always returned when they got too sick or the disease became too obvious, making outside life unbearable. My avowing that I would recover and leave and go home was met with great skepticism from the old, coldhearted gentleman.

My heart sank to a new low at the melancholy prospect of never returning to my home. I also thought then as I did later that it was rather cruel of Mr. Sellew to give that information to me. Why couldn't I be given something more encouraging to think about?

I was in prison for life, I thought, and my only crime was that of being sick. That wasn't fair. The place didn't look like a prison, quite the contrary, but not all prisons look like prisons.

Other kids were noticed clamoring around into the canteen, ordering cokes, 7ups, and strawberry sodas. I had never heard of any of those things, but everybody there seemed to really enjoy them. I found out that it cost five cents for one of these treats. Mother had given me a dollar for buying stamps and stationery, and I wondered if I dared spend a nickel on a soft drink.

Carefully considering it, I came to the conclusion that if Mom had been there and I had made the request, she probably would have granted my wish.

Watching the others, I coveted a strawberry soda most of all. It was such a pretty red, and everybody had a red tongue after they drank it. I bravely made the purchase and had a strange reaction to carbonated water and bittersweet flavor unknown to me. It was enjoyable, even the funny feeling in the nose and the tingling pinpoints of my tongue.

Feeling a little better after my new taste of soda pop, I started back to the house where I lived. There were bicycles everywhere, and everybody seemed to have one. Then I wondered how one would go about obtaining one of these and decided to find out as soon as possible.

On my arrival at the house, Pop Smith was sitting in his accustomed place on the porch, with his big wad of tobacco neatly tucked in his cheek. I eagerly approached him, asking how one went about getting a bike. I thought perhaps they were provided by the federal government, like everything else at Carville, but, alas, this was not true.

Pop Smith came up with a good idea. I could buy myself a bike if I got a job and paid for it! What jobs were available that I could do was another problem.

After a good bit of conversation, Pop again came up with a good idea. I could have the job of raising the flag each morning and taking it down each evening. The job paid a dollar a month. Some more discussion followed and the deal was consummated.

As time went by, I warmed up to the people there. I like Pop Smith and Sister Agnes especially. She encouraged me to take care of my health and gave hope of my eventual return home. I even grew to like the boys who had made me feel so uncomfortable on my first day there. It kind of made me feel accepted when I realized that the things they said were like the good-natured kidding from my pals back in school I had missed for so long. Mr. Sellew seemed more and more friendly to me. Although our first encounter had been a bit grim, I decided that, in being candid, he was actually being kind.

The people were nice; the place was nice. It was like eating a piece of pie with sand in it. You liked the taste but you didn't like what you were chewing on. Or it was like having a fly swimming around in your bowl of cream. *I was still sick!*

However, finally I began to feel more relaxed, once I settled into the routine of Carville life. I became more aware of the opportunities there, the prospect of making new friendships, though I reflected that the friends I really wanted were at home. I did, however, feel less confined than previously.

A few weeks after I took the job of raising and lowering, the flag, good old Pop Smith had a real surprise for me. He had bought a good used bike for two dollars and fifty cents.

He asked me if I would like to buy it from him. The terms would be twenty-five cents per month for ten months if I agreed.

Agree, I did. This was one of the proudest moments of my life and one of the happiest. Never before had I ever owned anything so expensive and useful. More important, I was paying for it myself with money earned. This was indeed a red-letter day for me.

Unfortunately, and I had not even considered this fact until this moment of proud ownership, I realized that I didn't know how to ride a bike. Happily, instead of returning it to him with a mournful tear in my eyes, saying I couldn't have a bike because I didn't know how to ride it, I learned to ride the thing. It was an imperceptible victory that I wasn't even aware of, but a victory nonetheless. Unable to wait another second for bicycle-riding lessons, I was determined to teach myself to balance and go. Pop Smith told me about a dirt road I could practice on, because, with all the other bike traffic, it would be too dangerous on the established paths. It was agreed that I would walk the bike to the practice area and walk it back until it had been determined that I was proficient enough to turn loose on the world.

The bike was obediently walked to the dirt road, and I proceeded to practice. With no one to help steady the thing, more than the usual share of problems were encountered in my attempts, and the air was blue with expletives, uttered at top voice, at the frustrations being encountered, but I kept on trying, more determined than ever to master this new skill.

With my vivid imagination, I thought of myself as a cowboy with a bucking bronco. Like a successful cowboy, I tamed the bronco, but not until more time was spent in the air and on the ground than on the bicycle. But after a lot of trying, became able to control the bike at all times.

Elated, I rode back to the cabin to tell Pop Smith the exciting news. How proud he would be upon seeing me pedaling so well, with everything under control, I thought, but I was in for a surprise.

He had given me explicit instructions about walking the bike to and from the practice area. The ability to operate the bike didn't bring with it automatic knowledge of safety rules and techniques. This he told me in emphatic and no uncertain terms.

When he was sure he had made himself clear, Pop Smith turned the conversation to other subjects. As was the case so many others who worked with and taught the young, I knew better than to belabor a point once it had been made.

After that conversation, I took the bike out often, but was more careful about the way I got to and from my destination.

As proficiency grew, I took more and longer rides around the compound, visiting the places I liked best. These rides also served the useful purpose of releasing pent-up feelings of frustration and anger.

On one of my rides I ventured to the front of the ground, where I had seen the white benches encircling the big shade trees. There I met a young couple who appeared to be extremely devoted to one another, but who also were very friendly and told me about more things that were available to the patients.

I learned about a screened-in pavilion where all sorts of social activities were held and learned about dances and other recreations taking place there, all was catered lavishly by the dinning-room personnel.

I, however, continued to resist even the most prodigious efforts to make me feel a part of the community there. Just when I would be welcome in a new situation that was of interest to me, I would make a tentative step in that direction, only to pull back because this wasn't the real home where I wanted to be.

Mom wrote often. Her letters would report on matters at home, and I read them avidly. The people who had shunned the family when they learned of my illness had never reestablished contact with them but had remained aloof. An occasional visitor would come to the farm, but the visits were stilted and short. Instructions and reminders about prayers and religion abounded in these epistles, and in perusing them, I was sure I could read between the lines. Knowing that I was responsible for the grief and privation that my family had suffered served to further inhibit any active participation in the activities that were on every side.

I would read and reread those messages from home, giving new meanings to each word I read, going on flights of fancy at each new interpretation. Most young men my age, couldn't wait to get away from the restrictions of home life. It would have been a bit odd for me to have this idea about my home had my physical condition of ten years' duration not existed. During all this constant thinking of home and family, I didn't think about the rest of the community and the way that part of my life had been. I would blame myself for my family's plight, but still wanted to be only there.

Between the long and frequent bike rides, I would haunt Sister Agnes's office. I was so devoted to my guiding angel and treasured her words of encouragement as though they were pearls from heaven. She would make inquiries as to my health, appetite, and activities, always commenting on the improvement in my physical appearance, which had been drastic. Sometimes Sister would ask me why I was there at her office, and I would give some stammering excuse to justify my presence.

The truth of the matter was that I adored Sister Agnes, much the way I adored Mom, and though this correlation never occurred to me, Sister was certainly aware of it, and the situation was not new to her or any other person in her position. She never bruised my feelings, for I was cooperative in my treatment program and she knew that her encouragement was desperately needed and important to my adjustment period.

On one of my frequent visits to see her, I learned that the patients were allowed ten days' vacation every six months, but we had to pay for and arrange transportation both ways and find our own driver. It was a double-edged situation. On the one hand, I was ecstatic with the prospect of going back home and seeing my family, but on the other hand, where in the world would the money come from? This was a real poser and cause of considerable thinking and worrying for me.

A few days after this intelligence had been gleaned from Sister Agnes, I was approached by Mr. Derf Tims, who was the manager of the canteen. Mr. Tims informed me that he had noticed me and was impressed with the good manners and respect I showed to my elders, which was so much a part of my personality. Because of that and other things that he found impressive, he offered me the position of courtesy clerk at the canteen. He went on to outline the duties of the position, which were many, and finished the description by saying that the position paid thirty-five dollars per month.

I couldn't believe my ears. Such a salary was unbelievably outrageous, and I decided without any further consideration that whatever the job entailed, I would be cheerful and efficient, for this, indeed, was a means for which the ends were justified.

I would just think of the money piling up sky high, dollar upon dollar! It wouldn't take any time at all to put away enough money to go home and be with those whom I held most dear. I accepted the job at once and began work the very next day.

I worked from 7:00 A.M. until 1:00 P.M. Even though I was the shyest of people, I became an enthusiastic entrepreneur, both dispensing the treats and displaying an engaging and friendly disposition with equal enthusiasm. I became a skilled soda-jerk and part-time fry cook of the indigestible fast foods that the customers were especially fond of. I even withstood the sometimes unkind references to my heavy accent and inability to understand precisely what was demanded of me by the customers. Each day I became a little more able to cope with these extreme frustrations.

I still had a couple of months to go before I was eligible to go home for my vacation, so I was extremely diligent and perspicacious in the handling of my earnings. The time was speeding by surprisingly quickly. No longer was each day an endless period to be endured. With my new activities and my time better and more effectively organized, the special day for which I had been praying so fervently was soon upon me.

Mr. Krub, the driver, pulled up in front of the hospital early that Sunday morning. Everyone's luggage was ready, and we eagerly piled into the automobile for the trip to our respective destinations.

In my case, though the shortest possible route was taken, the original trip was retraced. The trip was uneventful except for when we passed through Kaplan, where my fondest memories had been of school and Gleanda. I was surprised that my cherished memories were so acutely awakened. I just hadn't been aware that they were quite as dormant as they had become. In passing through Kaplan, my memories were certainly dormant no more. We passed within blocks of Dr. Latina's office though the recollections of that fateful visit were not in any way the same as those of my school days.

I thought again of Gleanda. How I wished I could again look into those beautiful eyes or have her ask if she could dip her pen into my inkwell or do any of the other silly but painfully remembered little things I associated with this little girl.

I bet that by now she was the prettiest and the most popular young lady in school. She was most certainly the smartest, as well. I wondered how many more honors she had accumulated since she had so impressively eliminated all her competition in that first spelling bee. If I should walk up to her after all this time, would she remember me? Could she recognize me? Would she welcome me with all the affection I had had for her for so many years? I was sure she would. Such a perfect human being, so smart, so beautiful, so understanding, just couldn't possibly be anything else than I had remembered her. I felt that I was being unjust to her to a certain point. Most certainly, she was much better than I recalled, and I even felt guilty for doubting that she would remember me or recognize me or in any way fail to reciprocate my love, If anything, she probably had been waiting for my return, spurning all hopeful suitors, faithfully and chastely. She would be Evangeline forever searching for Gabriel, waiting, and remaining true. It would never matter to dear Gleanda/Evangeline that I/Gabriel was in a holy war for my life. She would enter a convent before she would surrender that loving memory. Should she meet me again before entering a convent, she would risk contagion before she would lose her love again.

The old jerky road took us closer to home. We passed through Cassinade, where I had first started school, where more memories abounded, both of early school days and of Gleanda.

There was the old cemetery where those dear, innocent twin baby girls of Uncle Yas's lay sleeping alongside other relatives I fondly recalled.

We passed the homes of my friends from school as we neared our destination.

We passed the red-and-white cattle, so familiar to me, grazing contentedly on either side of the road, as the road itself became more and more difficult because the monsoon rains had done their usual damage, each year the roads remained unrepaired, the ruts having been enhanced by those big, steel wagon wheels.

Mr. Krub interrupted my reveries with "Where the hell do you live, anyway? Can we go the rest of the way in the car or will we have to go by mule?"

I was snapped back to life, because, at this point, we were coming onto the old road that led directly to the house, directly to the only home I had ever known or wanted to know. After a right turn, I jumped out of the vehicle, opened the wire gate, and we were homeward bound.

Finally, it came into view. There was the lone figure of one of the twins standing watch. Within seconds, the word had been spread, and as we approached I saw the whole family congregated on the front porch.

I was finally back home. Words, hugs, and every kind of affectionate and loving greeting engulfed me. Everyone greeted me but Rip. Tears of joy streamed from my mother's eyes, and the chaos at the front gate to the house was something to behold. Some of the loose boards on the old porch still needed nails. Mr. Krub deposited my luggage when I got out of the car at the gate, and Maloon dutifully carried it to the house for me. Mr. Krub, having other deliveries to make, waved good-bye. I almost missed it, but didn't fail to return it, and he turned around and went on to his destination.

After the initial hysteria and greetings on my return home, the family walked the rest of the distance to the house in comparative silence, unable to adequately express their emotions, silence taking the place of words.

Home at last, home at last, Thank God Almighty, I'm home at last, I thought.

Once inside and comfortably seated in the living room, everybody wanted to know all about what had been happening at Carville and no detail should be omitted. As I had written home faithfully and frequently, there was very little news I could add, but the family never tired of hearing about my new adventures again and again, asking questions at each telling.

Finally, a little embarrassed at being the one doing all the talking, I asked questions about what had been going on at home while I was away.

My mother gave me a description of what had happened at home, and very little of what she told me was news, as she, too, had done quite a bit of letter writing, dictating her French to Maloon, but I wanted to hear about it anyway. I mainly wanted to hear her voice again and was not disappointed. A garrulous person on her worst days, she was even more verbose on this occasion.

The old matriarch concluded her colorful narrative by obliquely mentioning the fact that there hadn't been any fish on the table since I went away. She also added that my fishing lines were where I had left them, just beyond the second bend in the river, hanging from the tree to keep dry.

I certainly didn't need any encouragement in that direction. Fishing and hunting, my favorite of all pursuits, were things I had dreamed of doing ever since I went away, but particularly since I had learned that I would come home for a visit. It made me feel good, however, that my mom was encouraging me in doing what I wanted to do so badly. I would also be making a contribution to the family. I was really the only one other than mother who had a passion for fishing.

The conversation turned to school and the things happening there. I would never, ever in a million years let my brothers, sisters, or parents know that what I wanted to hear about was my beloved Gleanda, and unfortunately, nothing about her was mentioned. My brothers reported mainly on things that had gone wrong. I never tired of hearing about school, as I had been a good student while attending, not counting when I became ill, and wanted all the news, good or bad.

My older brother Maloon discreetly related the incidents that brought about the discredit or downfall of other less obedient and careful students than himself. When I learned of some of these antics, I rolled with laughter.

Warming to the subject, Darbee had stories of his own to tell. Unfortunately, he was the subject of some of the derring-do, and as he enthusiastically unfolded tale after tale, he inadvertently mentioned a couple of paddlings he had received from teachers. Upon hearing of these infractions, Mom, who had been listening and laughing along with everyone else, perked up her ears. One of the rules of the family was that under no circumstances should any of the children be disobedient to the teachers. If it should become necessary for a teacher to administer corporal punishment to any of Mother's brood, she had a bonus for whoever it might be at home. So there, in the midst of all the gaiety and laughters, the razor strop was once again called into action and administered to a very unhappy Darbee.

My brother's sidelong glances in my direction seemed to be saying that I had somehow been responsible. Even though I felt sorry for my brother, I couldn't but remember all those times when Maloon and I had had a taste of the strop when Darbee had brought one of his news flashes to our mom. I, in typical schoolboy fashion, reflected upon the fact that teachers were sometimes wrong. I remember a few occasions when, acting on spurious information or downright lies, a teacher had administered a ruler to a student. I recalled once when I had had the honor of being spanked myself. I had always felt that the teacher had been pretty mean for not having believed my story or excuse given to justify my actions; the fact that I had lied was notwithstanding. The teacher was blamed for not keeping better control of her temper.

My sister Joan, also had tales to tell, but, like Maloon, she was discreet. Joan was a wit and the family comedienne. Nearly everything she said, whether seriously or in jest, had a way of tickling everyone's funnybone. This was true even if she made a simple remark about the weather or some other innocent subject; it would come out outrageously funny.

This was such a warm and happy reunion for me. Everybody had been so dearly missed, and now I was with them and experiencing all the laughter and love that we shared among ourselves.

Mr. Joseph LeBeaux had a few stories to tell about his faux pas, too. The long hours that he worked in isolation didn't give rise to a lot of things to relate in reference to his own particular errors. I reasoned that if my father made any gross mistakes, there was never anyone there to know about it, so why should he admit that they took place at all? Sly fox, my father.

What a sumptuous supper we had that evening! My mother had cooked all the old favorites, which had been so badly missed at Carville. I couldn't express my happiness and contentment at being back home. It was like slipping into an old pair of worn-out shoes. It just felt so good and so right. If I hadn't been so happy to see my family, I might have felt guilty about it.

The next morning, I watched as my brothers started down the long path to the school-bus stop. Again I felt the old pang of regret, knowing that I would never walk that path again.

My mom had been anxiously waiting to talk to me alone. She asked more questions about Carville and how I was getting along there. Being so close to Mother and loving her as I did, I just didn't want to tell her how unhappy I had been, especially at first. A bright picture was painted, as I told her all about my many new friends and the numerous activities in which I participated and once again gave the details of how I had been able to purchase a bike and about the job I had for the purpose. We went into greater detail about my position at the canteen that had enabled me to make this return visit. It was so good to be with Mom again that every word I uttered was carefully edited, as I did not want to make her unhappy.

I went so far as to tell her that with my new job and everything else that I had to do, hunting and fishing were scarcely missed. After another cup of our supreme Louisiana coffee and a big hug and kiss from Mom, I went outside to look around.

As I walked all around that familiar area, everything I saw brought memories to me, some sweet, some bitter. The memories were very strong, and a glance would bring back years and years of episodes in a flash.

I went down to the river and found my fishing lines as I had left them. I looked around, found bait, baited the hooks, set the lines, then hastily departed.

I was afraid to fall any more in love with all this than I already was, because it would be all the harder to leave. I wanted to not experience the pains of remembering the things I loved most with the same intensity I had experienced when first arriving at Carville.

As I started back to the house, I realized I had made a technical error when I told Mother I didn't have time to miss fishing and hunting. What a stupid thing to tell her! Of all the people in the world, my mother, above all, knew how much I cared about these pursuits. They were the only things that held me together during those years of unhappiness and exclusion before I went to Carville. I had just wanted to spare her feelings but I knew that I hadn't really fooled her at all.

Mother had a way of getting things out of people, one way or another, and I decided there had been too much deceit already. I thought of all that time at school telling those outright lies about my worsening condition, of the stories I had made up to explain my constant presence around Sister Agnes's office, and of other times that my conscience wouldn't let me forget. I was determined to tell Mother the entire truth and then console her if I could.

When I went back into the house, I did just that. Judging from the expression on her face, as I unfolded my unhappy story of the way I had really felt when I arrived at Carville, she wasn't really surprised. Even though her face was continuously bathed with the usual tears, I knew I was doing the right thing.

Even the hurt and humiliation at hearing unkind references to my countrified behavior and to my ignorance of the most rudimentary operation of the appliances, which the other boys took for granted, were confessed.

Once I got started, the words just wouldn't stop. I kept on talking and talking, and finally there was nothing left to say about my many frustrations at moving to Carville.

Unknown to me, I had just told Mother things I had never mentioned to her before and, by doing so, experienced a great emotional catharsis. Before leaving home, I had remained silent for years about the way I felt, and now I was speaking openly for the first time about my own feelings.

When the subject of my unhappiness was finally exhausted, I told Mother about the beloved Sister Agnes. I talked about our many visits together and of the spiritual strength she had that she had imparted to me. Many phrases of encouragement and comfort were quoted that Sister had addressed to me, and I told Mother how alike she and Sister Agnes were.

When Mother was told about my reaction to the first encounter

I had had with Sister, a sparkle of mirth found its way through the tears that by now were generously flowing. I was just being candid and forthright, and my mom was experiencing great comfort, especially when I spoke of Sister Agnes. After all, Mom's favorite subject next to her family was religion, and she was not only pleased to know that I was so close to a holy person, but that I was attending mass, going to confession, and receiving Holy Communion regularly. She treasured this relationship between her son and the good nun more than any riches. She agreed wholeheartedly with what Sister had told me about prayers and faith, though she thought she could never have expressed it so eloquently.

This exchange between Mother and me marked the first adult conversation I ever had. Come what may, in the future I would look at things in a much more mature manner. Above all, I had the important resolve that come what may, I would come back home, and come back cured.

Throughout my visit home, Mother and I would have conversations each day on the things that Sister Agnes had had to say. Her faith and knowledge of God was something that Mom shared to the very core of her being, and though not as knowledgeable on all aspects of that faith as Sister Agnes, she appreciated the information I had to offer and readily accepted any new pieces of information. More important still was the fact that her son had a dear and loving friendship with one of the finest people he could ever find on the face of the earth. If she couldn't care for her son herself, she couldn't imagine another person to whom his care could be entrusted, a person better qualified and better able to give him what he required, than Sister Agnes. In her daily prayers, Mom thanked God for Sister Agnes and prayed that I would never have to be separated from this blessed nun.

During my brief visit, the time seemed to be racing by me like the world was hurrying up. It hardly seemed possible that time would slip by so fast. Days and nights just seemed to all come together.

I would fish and Mom would usually accompany me. I, in turn, would help with meal preparation and anything else around the house that needed doing.

With all the activites that Mom and I shared, it was in my private moments that my thoughts would turn to my old school chums. I would look down the road in hopes of seeing a friendly face coming my way. This happened almost daily, though it was never mentioned. I would think of my old friends and wonder why, when we lived so close to them, they didn't drop by for even a quick hello. The road was always empty when I looked, first this way and then that.

Even more than my friends I hoped to see lovely Gleanda. I knew that if she had any notion that I was back home, she would find a way to come by to see me, if only for a moment. The deep love that I knew she shared with me would compel her to see me while I was home. I would dream of just one stolen moment with my love. The thought of just the touch of her fingertips upon me or her wave as she approached my house was an exquisite pain to me. I would imagine all sorts of chance or planned meetings with her, and when at the end of my visit when those visits had not occurred, I treasured the golden memories of the fictions I had invented.

I further reflected that it would have made Mom so happy if some of my friends had come by to see me.

As this visit was beginning to wind down and the time was nearing for my departure, I tried to spend even more time with Mom, who was beginning to cry more and more in anticipation of my return to Carville. How I wished that I was not the source of her worry and unhappiness. I was well aware of how desolate I had been when I had to leave my family and knew it was much worse for my highly emotional mother. She had been so happy at my return and so determined to make my visit a happy one that she had kept a little secret of her own from me. It wasn't until my persistent questions could no longer be evaded that she finally told me through an ocean of tears.

After my departure to Carville, my loyal, beloved pet had moped around and didn't want to eat or chase rabbits or do anything. Rip was mourning my leaving just as my mother was. He would run to the front gate whenever he heard anyone coming, only to return sad and disappointed. Then one day he had followed Dad to town, probably hoping to find his master there. On that trip, a wagon had run over Rip, killing him. My parents deeply mourned the lost of my pet, as he had been something of a comfort in spite of his obvious unhappiness at the disappearance of his master.

I hadn't asked about my pet chicken. I had seen at once that the little chick who had taken me as her surrogate mother so long ago and continued her allegiance through adulthood was nowhere to be found. I figured that my little pet had stopped laying and wasn't pulling her weight around the barnyard and knew from past experience what that meant. If you were a chicken on that farm and got lazy, you were moved to the top of the list of those earmarked for Mom's stew pot. Not wanting to bring on any more guilty tears, I just didn't ask about the chicken, but she hadn't been forgotten.

As time grew short, I went out to the pasture we sometimes shared with our landlord, in search of my goats, Petite and Billy.

It took a bit of searching, but I found Petite first. She was just as gentle as always and responded warmly when I put my arms around her neck in a big hug. She hadn't forgotten me! What a relief that was. Billy, on the other hand, was another story. Being the more daring of the pair, he had wandered far and wide and, like me, loved the freedom that being on the range offered. When I finally located him and called him he remembered me but stayed aloof, almost daring me to catch up with him. He played the little game out as long as he could, then, with a leap and a bleat, came toward me and his former teammate, Petite. Reluctantly, he permitted himself to be petted and talked to, but seemed to be ready to bolt any moment.

I remained with the goats awhile, then turning slowly toward the house, bade them good-bye, and hoped that they would remain free and safe in a place they love. I didn't want to get too close to the pets, as I knew I would be leaving soon. *But I will be back*, I thought. *I will be back, and I will be well.*

The air of the countryside smelled sweet and fresh as I walked through the woods back home. I could see from a distance that

Mother was working industriously in the kitchen, probably fixing supper. It was getting late, but I didn't hurry. I relished the sights of the land and was trying to absorb as much of it as I could before going back to Carville.

Mother was crying even more now in anticipation of my departure. There wasn't anything to be done about this. She didn't seem to know any other way to react to the frustration and regretted that her son was ill and that he would be leaving soon. But just about when she was almost completely overcome, she would remember Sister Agnes and her wise and sacred words of encouragement to me and would be somewhat consoled.

When the day finally arrived for me to go, another crowd assembled at the edge of the yard. There had been no other visits. This time, however, there were fewer people. It was still a silent crowd that came to supervise my departure.

Remembering the last time I had left and my humiliation, I made no effort to get close to anyone or to extend my hand. Mom, of course was disconsolate, but I was able to hug and kiss her goodbye, pull away from her, and get into the car. When the car left, she again tried to follow it, but not quite with the same intensity as before. I watched her as long as I could, but when we went around the curve again, everything disappeared from view—Mom, the farm, the neighbors, everything. I thought to myself that it was as though they had never been there. I felt as if I were waking up after a dream.

I knew what was ahead of me on the trip back to Carville. First, was to pass the little schoolhouse where I had started school and where Gleanda and I had sat, one behind the other, from the very beginning. The same memories of the friends I had had and the games we had played came back to me.

We drove on and came to Kaplan. That was where Gleanda lived. The whole town took on a different meaning because of her. It was *her* town. Things there were better and nicer because *she* lived there. I kept a constant lookout all the while we drove through it on the chance that I might spy her somewhere thereabouts. She was not to be seen anywhere, but it was still *her* town. We drove on, but I thought, *I'll be back and I'll be well.*

My appearance was vastly improved after a time back at the hospital. My hands looked normal, and there was only the slightest trace of swelling of my face. I was becoming surer and surer that my days at Carville were numbered and that it wouldn't be very long before I could go home, completely well.

It wasn't time yet. I got sick. The flag was still faithfully raised and lowered each day and I worked in the canteen, but was forced to spend more and more time in bed.

I bought a radio so I could listen to my favorite country-western music while I spent so much time in my room. This weakness was short-lived, however, and soon I was back on the job again, happy as ever. *Just a minor setback*, I thought.

One day out of the blue, I had a reaction. At that time nobody knew if the reaction was due to the drugs that were taken daily or to the progress of the disease itself. A reaction wasn't anything new to the patients at Carville. Everybody seemed to have a reaction from time to time, some more than others, but this was the first time I had such an experience. My arms, hands, legs, torso, and face were covered with what looked for all the world like cherry size, flaming red marbles. This was accompanied by a raging fever and pain throughout my entire body. I had to be hospitalized immediately, as I was far too ill to do the least thing to care for myself. Fortunately, the attack lasted only about a week, but took its toll. I suffered a terrific weight loss. I was awfully weak, not only because of the weight loss, but because I had been hit hard. It was necessary that I be careful during my recuperation from all this and take things slow and easy while I regained my strength. This episode didn't do much to improve my disposition, either, as it was interfering with my plans to get well and go home.

Then there were more reactions. The will to live would come and go. When it came, it reinforced the courage to continue with the battle. When it did not, the fight became more difficult. I tried to get sympathy from the patients, but nobody would listen. They had troubles of their own.

I was to learn as much as possible about the disease that plagued me. As with almost anything, the more information one has, the better able he or she is to cope with the situation and cooperate in the treatment of it and, hopefully, avoid the most destructive of all attitudes, that of self-pity.

One of the most prominent pieces of information I was to learn was that I should always refer to the disease by its proper medical name, Hansen's disease, after the Norwegian scientist who had first identified the bacteria that causes it. He had also been a part of an enormous effort of members of the medical community, the patients, and other informed people to do everything possible to give the information that they had as to the nature of the illness and its treatment, an effort that has gradually grown in scope, but not nearly enough, among the general public.

The advent of the fourth decade of the twentieth century brought with it some new things at Carville. An extensive renewal and expansion of the facilities was undertaken, much to the approval and appreciation of the patients, not to mention the staff. Everything was rebuilt and refurbished in the lastest fashion. Not only were the accommodations updated, but the laboratory facilities were made more efficient and effective through the installation of every new diagnostic tool.

We all felt that despite the fact that we were constantly shown every consideration in our treatment and comfort, there was more caring still from the great world outside our confines.

Patients kept dying. We'd joke about the gravedigger, Chief, standing around with his shovel in his hands waiting for one of us to go so he could make himself a few bucks. Although this was unconfirmed, the life expectancy of the patients, as Dr. Latina had said, was probably about a true five years.

The early forties also brought about a creative and innovative patient, Mr. Stanly Stein, with a new idea that was to grow and flourish. He founded a publication called *The Star*. In it were contributions from the patients, and, more important, from the physicians, detailing the latest treatments being investigated as well as new drugs that seemed to be either just around the corner or possbily closer than that. Patients' awareness was greatly enhanced, and the beginning of the age of mutual cooperation in the treatment of diseases between patients and health care professionals was inaugurated. We were educated in more detail about our disease and were reminded never to use the word leprosy in reference to it. That prestigious magazine, *The Star,* is still being published and has attracted worldwide attention because of its efforts. Though Mr. Stein died later, he was succeeded by a competent Mr. Louis Boudreaux. The magazine managed to overcome the detrimental setback of the loss of Mr. Stein and has continued to meet the needs and demands placed upon it. It is of note that Mr. Stein was blind and, in spite of that, he never relented in his effort to insure the success of his venture. In his book *The Power of Positive Thinking,* Norman Vincent Peale said of the magazine: "a great human document with startling evidence of the power of the human spirit to overcome adversity." Dr. John R. Trautman, director of the National Hansen's Disease Research Center, in Carville, Louisiana, said of the publication: "This book carries so poignantly the message to which Stanly Stein dedicated himself and which *The Star* so ably continued to convey through its pages."

This fine man touched many many lives with his courage and foresight, and his influence is still felt by those who knew him, of whom I was one.

In that same year, something new came into my life (other than new symptoms of Hansen's disease). I was attending a baseball game one evening when I looked up and beheld who I considered to be the most attractive and exciting young lady I had ever seen. The impact was something like being hit by a runaway freight train.

I saw beautiful green eyes that appeared to be spotted with tiny snowflakes. The woman behind the eyes, wearing a gorgeous red bandanna tied beneath her chin, made my heart sing. I was instantly besotted by her and mute, as usual. My mind immediately raced into all sorts of wild plans to make her acquaintance and, at the same time, how to forestall any and all competition from all other men from sixteen to sixty, or maybe a hundred and sixty. I was determined that this beautiful woman must be mine. Since my entire previous romantic involvement had been with my memories and fantasies of Gleanda that had taken place solely in my imagination, I was not completely prepared to begin my courtship of this glamorous lovely. My strategy was carefully planned.

Having failed to attract the attention of the young lady that evening, I waited a couple of weeks, learning all I could about her. I tried what I felt was the perfect plan. Her name was Maria, and she was from Zapata, Texas. She was of Mexican origin and had all the qualities and beauty of her native country.

In the dining room during lunch, I chose a position in close proximity to Maria and burst into a loud song, singing the currently popular "South of the Border, Down Mexico Way," a favorite of mine that always elicited exciting and romantic visions in my mind and therefore, I reasoned, would accomplish the same with Maria. Wrong!

That young woman couldn't have cared less about me and my song, and I might as well have been invisible. Smarting from the failure of my grand gesture, I sneaked away, humiliated beyond description, but undeterred. I would think of something else.

If Boothe Tarkington had heard about or known me, D. J. LeBeaux, the chronicles of my love and pursuit of Maria would be required reading in literature classes throughout the land.

In an effort to demonstrate my intellectual prowess, I secured the dictionary, finding long and exotic words with which to impress Maria when the fateful moment came when we were to speak. I assiduously paid attention to my grooming and wardrobe, being careful to coordinate every item of clothing for impeccable matching. My thick mop of hair was another matter and now seemed to require extra, but rewarding, efforts to coif it perfectly. Each of these and other things I undertook in order to make myself irresistible to Maria. They became a daily ritual, sometimes requiring nearly the entire day. Still, Maria hadn't noticed me.

Then I started shadowing her. I would stay at what I felt was a discreet distance and observe her every move as often as I could. I would turn green with jealously if she sat next to any male, young or old, whether they were together or not. I would visualize duels during which I would fell all opponents in order to win the fair Maria's hand. She remained unaware of my presence, even when I stood in the back of the theater like a mannequin with its feet glued to the floor, watching every move she made.

Whenever Maria stopped in the canteen, I would go out of my way to be courteous to her, demonstrating my charm and attentiveness to her every want and need. Once I went so far as to ask her for the money to pay for her purchase. That request was met with a fiery retort, as she had fully intended to pay me, but hadn't gotten the money from her purse quickly enough. She had a way with words that might have discouraged a less determined young man, but not me.

On my trusty bicycle, I would drive pass the house in which she lived. I wanted to check upon her companions and whomever she spoke to. Many times I thought I would casually drive up to the porch where she would be sitting and casually engage her in a conversation carefully prepared, on my part. On each occasion, I would start in that direction, only to lose courage at the very last minute and ride straight past, eyes straight ahead, for all the world as if I were rehearsing for the Olympic bicycle race.

The thought occurred to me that perhaps the best approach would be a direct one: just walk right up to her and start talking and get to know her. But this was impossible. I was sure that if I tried it, she would not only reject me but probably tell me never to come back and laugh at me. That was definitely out. By now, I was beginning to run out of ideas and just had to find a way. I was beginning to be a bit self-conscious, wondering if anyone had noticed my attempts, however futile, to make the acquaintance and gain the favor of Maria. I really wished that she would have only other young ladies for friends and only me for a sweetheart.

Maybe if I appeared detached and disinterested, that might do the trick. I knew well how Mother would go crazy trying to please me whenever I pouted and sulked. Then I decided that that is what I would do, knowing it was certain to work on Maria. Maria, it turned out, was not only not my mother but nothing like Mom in that respect. What could I try next?

Right in the middle of all my posturing and planning, the other patients and I got word of a wonderful new drug from abroad that was reputed to be the answer to all our hopes and dreams. Being a new drug (diptheria toxoid), it was used on a strictly volunteer basis. Needless to say, there was no shortage of volunteers. Nobody at Carville wanted to spend the rest of his life there, and it was almost unanimously decided to give the new drug a try.

The treatment commenced forthwith. After a few months of treatments, a couple of things happened. One group of patients showed no improvement at all and had one reaction after another, the episodes becoming longer, more severe, and more frequent. Those in this group would spend months in the hospital, too ill to move and so miserable and disappointed as to give up hope, in some cases. The recovery from this disaster was protracted and difficult, with lingering symptoms that seemed never to completely leave us.

I was among the group that suffered the severe reactions, and my recovery, like the others' was very, very slow. I was gradually regaining a bit of strength as Christmas neared.

The nuns had a gala Christmas party planned for us youngsters. It was always a lot of fun for us, but this year, in particular, it was special because it marked the end of the ghastly episode with the disappointing new drug. We young boys and girls were in a festive mood that day and maybe a bit feisty at being able to do something different and feel more alive.

A girl by the name Nenne and I, along with some of our cohorts, decided to make the evening even merrier by entering into a criminal conspiracy. It was a well-planned and carefully executed theft, the subject of which was Sister Cathy's bottle of whiskey. This added a further note on intrigue, as it was strictly forbidden to have any alcoholic beverages on government property, except for beer, which had to be consumed in the canteen.

With each coconspirator doing his assigned task, Nenne pilfered the aforementioned bottle. Sister Cathy had received special dispensation from the medical director for said bottle, only because it was to be used on this special occasion for the eggnog and punch at the annual Christmas party. This illegal action was accompanied with a lot of "shhs" and deadpan faces on the part of us felons, who were fully aware of the gravity of our dastardly deed.

Once the whiskey had been obtained and nearly everyone had gotten a quick snort, I drank more than a spoonful. It made me cough a little and put a silly smile on my face. Then the contraband liquid was neatly tucked away next door, in a filing cabinet drawer by smart Nenne.

The disappearance of the bottle of firewater had its problems.

We made Sister Cathy feel as if she were unjustly questioning a group of the most pure and innocent children, children who under no circumstances would even dream of undertaking a deed so vile. For some strange reason, however, almost suddenly inquisitions concerning the reprehensible deed was dropped and no further mention of it was made.

We thieves shared not only a sigh of relief, but a secret satisfaction at our success at stealing and, above all, our own acting abilities.

As the party progressed, spirits ran high, as it were, and revelry escalated. I had never before been so confident or loquacious. As a matter of fact, most of the revelers showed some of the same self-confidence when who should appear, albeit a bit late for the occasion, but the glamorous Maria!

Unhampered by my usual social ineptitude, I was quite able to engage the young woman in productive conversation. I learned all sorts of things about her, and all the things learned served to reinforce my already great love for and admiration of this treasured prize. I was so very careful not to betray the shameful action that had taken place prior to her arrival at the party. Surely, had she known of any of it, she would have been shocked and probably would have reported the entire episode, out of sheer honesty and revulsion at such terrible behavior on the part of the group who had perpetrated the securing of Sister Cathy's bottle.

Maria's pristine goodness and purity were almost overwhelming to me. The mere fact that Maria and I were conversing made my head reel. It opened my life, I found out that nervously, in love, I could still converse, even braced by alcohol. If it weren't for the bottle of whiskey stolen from Sister Cathy, who knows all the things that might not have happened?

Not long after the Christmas party, there was a dance held in the huge new recreation hall and I had another chance to see Maria. I also got another chance to taste the liquor. Nenne, friend to all, had the firewater securely put away in her umbrella, hanging inside her closet, and was kind enough to pass the key to her room around, thus enabling us boys, traveling in twos or threes, to go to the designated place and have a few quick ones.

By the time that Maria came upon the scene, I was feeling no pains and was in the same outgoing frame of mind as I had been at the Christmas party. She was very friendly to me, and I had visions of dancing the night away with this sweet person.

Somehow, I was always able to grab defeat from the jaws of victory, and this time I committed a grand faux pas. In the middle of a lively jitterbug Maria and I were doing, I kicked Maria on the leg to the beat of "The Two O'clock Jump." There was a step where you kicked your right foot forward and then backward, and when I attempted this, my forward stroke hit her on the shin. I had spent literally hours alone in my room learning to be a good dancer to the sound of the radio, but the enthusiasm of the dance, the booze, and my excitement at being with Maria, had made me lose control. She was stunned by the agonizing pain of such an untimely and unfortunate accident and had to be physically assisted to her table amidst a great profusion of apologies from me. She was understanding, of course, but I wanted to die of embarrassment.

She showed self-possession and tact by moving to my table, where we spent the remainder of the evening, just talking and making a lot of eye contact. If I said or did anything else unseemly, she never betrayed it to me or anyone else. I had a reputation for being courteous and well mannered up until this time, but this night I was not at my best. I just couldn't believe that the whole place had witnessed the accident. In my heart, I felt that I was being judged harshly.

The following morning, I kept a sharp lookout for her. On her entrance into the dining room, at the appropriate time I slipped into line with her. She showed great pleasure at seeing me and told me how much she had enjoyed the previous evening, making no reference to the fact that I had been falling-down drunk. Again I was elated beyond reason. This was a dream come true.

It was at this time that I received devastating news from home. There had been a great flood, and the normally quiet river I loved so well had overflowed its banks, inundating the entire farm. The house where I happily spent my childhood years had been submerged up to its roof by the raging waters. The family had lost everything they had.

My family was evacuated to Kaplan, where they were fed and

clothed by the Red Cross. They stayed there for quite some time, as everyone waited for the floodwaters to subside. The Red Cross also provided the family with a few essentials when they returned to dig out the silt and try to clean the place up and put it in some kind of order. All their livestock and gardens and farm equipment were gone, and though they tried desperately to put things back together, it was no use. The decision was finally made to move to Kaplan for good and try some kind of steady employment.

When word got out of their decision to move, it was greeted rather warmly by the community, which had been less than cordial ever since my affliction had become known. They were permitted to purchase the house for a very modest sum. A house valued at about $2,000.00 was sold to them for $400.00, at payments of $10.00 a month. The generosity on the part of the landlord was rooted in practicality. It had been made clear to him that no one would ever live in that house and that if it were left there vacant, it probably would have to be burned to the ground in order to protect the unwary from the dreaded disease I had. My family then had this house moved to town.

None of this was easy for the family and me. It was a completely new life facing my family, one that none of them had ever imagined. All of them loved living on the farm and were afraid of the "city life" that they were now entering. I, on the other hand, had pinned my hopes and dreams of leaving Carville on returning to the farm, where I hoped to spend the rest of my life tending the crops and animals. Now there was no farm and no family there anymore. It was worse than a death in the family, and the loss was mourned. I always wondered what had become of my fishing lines and my goat cart and to what extent Billy and Petite had suffered before death came to them in the raging waters, after having hit trees in the swift waters pushed, scratched, and bruised, only to be left helpless. I also wondered about a marble I had tucked in a knothole underneath the house. It was all very unsettling.

Now I was forced to do some serious thinking and reevaluation of my goals and priorities and also forced to think and evaluate in a much more mature manner than I had done previously. My goals had always been to return to the security blanket of the farmland, my memories of which were somewhat distorted due to my nonacceptance of the way things really were.

The ambivalent feelings I had had for so many years were being placed out in front of me to judge and to resolve. I had always eschewed the responsibility of making decisions, but decisions were now being forced upon me. This time there was no fantasy world to turn to and no fictitious scenario to act out. Mother couldn't advise me or manipulate me anymore. In short, I was faced with the responsibility of becoming a man, with all its attendant responsibilities.

I finally came to grips with the fact that even if it had been feasible to return to the farm, I would have been no more welcome than I had been before my departure to Carville. That was the hardest thing for me to accept, but the acceptance finally came and with it a different kind of peace of mind, completely new to me.

During this melancholy time, something else was happening to me, so gradually that it was some time before I realized it. The new medication, Promin, that I had been taking seemed to have been doing the job. Almost before I knew it, the pains were gone along with the severe abdominal reactions I had experienced.

This turn of events was certainly a welcome one, coming as it did on the heels of the loss of home. I enjoyed the feeling of good health, and wanted it to continue.

The sweet Lorelei's song of life outside Carville was beckoning me and urging me to taste the freedom, to share in the life denied me for so many years. Thoughts of life outside the confines of Carville began to take on a new meaning. Even back-breaking work looked good to me. Most of all, I was healthy and looked fine. Gone were not only the pains, but the swelling and disfigurement of my face. Not a trace of discoloration remained. On the same positive note as the improvement of my health was my developing relationship with Maria. She had been at my side, offering encouragement and understanding during my deep unhappiness and grief at the loss of my home and at my family's suffering. She never pushed and never insisted or demanded, but, as a giving person, gave me the strength of her lovely soul and devout prayers. My awareness of the closeness and mutual affection that had developed between us was also gradual.

Probably because of my preoccupation with my family, or maybe just because I was becoming a mature adult, I somehow managed to stop doing myself harm by saying all the wrong things to her. I had now become able to transcribe my thoughts on paper, sending them to Maria. I still couldn't find the courage to tell her of my deepening love and devotion, but on other matters I was fairly eloquent.

One day, I came close to expressing my thoughts on paper, but stopped just short of telling her. Maria, being no fool, asked me exactly what my note meant. I told her that I wanted her to be my girl and that I loved her and wanted to spend the rest of my life with her.

I astonished myself with such a bold answer, but was even more astonished and ecstatic when she agreed to go steady. This was almost too much to accept at one time, but somehow I managed and didn't have the presence of mind to ruin the whole thing, as I had characteristically done on other occasions.

After a few weeks of courtship, she confessed her love to me. I just couldn't believe it, and there was no way to describe my elation at learning the news. After the initial shock had worn off, I began to detail the many years of loving from afar and the numerous ruses that I had devised in order to attract her attention. The smiles, laughter, and warm tears sealed our love, our mutual confessions to one another, the greatest prize being, the mutually shared love that was real and not imaginary.

The canteen had changed hands by now and was being operated by the Patients Federation. Because of my many years' experience working there, I was made manager. It was necessary that I learn all the details of management, including bookkeeping reading the invoices, et cetera. I mastered these skills in record time. My salary was also upgraded from $35.00 dollars per month to $150.00 per month. By the time of my resignation, some three years later, I had amassed savings of several thousand dollars.

During my on-the-job training in business administration, I wanted to set a wedding date with Maria. Together we could use the savings to establish a new life together outside the big fence of Carville.

Maria was responding equally well to the new course of treatment we were both receiving. She had always been beautiful, but by now was positively glowing. We would have long talks about what it would be like living on the "outside," both of us contributing to the goal which we were by now pursuing together.

When I made my final proposal of marriage to her, there was no hesitation on her part. Her immediate answer was "Yes," accompanied by a big kiss, my first as an adult. It was a tender moment, radiantly full of love, as we sat in the park under the famous oak trees with the white benches beneath. The mental image of the beautiful girl that beautiful day was to always remain with me, always fresh and never worn like a photograph. We spent hours discussing our wedding plans and other plans for the future. It was a time to explore, a time to dream, a time to set values.

Hospital regulations prevented the local priest, Father Rono, from performing the wedding ceremony, much to my and Maria's mutual disappointment. There were so many things we couldn't do there. We couldn't vote, couldn't utilize public transportation, couldn't spend time together in the women's dormitories, and couldn't get married.

So we had to revert to the underground. This movement had been established by some of the most daring patients who were willing to risk apprehension by the guards when going through the hole in the side of the barbed-wire fence or returning. It wasn't certain what the penalty of being caught might be. It was reasonable to assume that we wouldn't be shot or thrown into solitary confinement, but the rules were vigorously enforced and respected by most of the patients.

By means of this underground grapevine, Maria and I learned that there was a priest who would perform the ceremony and a doctor who would administer the physical tests required by law in order for us to obtain a marriage license.

Armed with this intelligence, Maria and I decided to take our vacations together at the same time. We had long since learned about securing transportation and saving for vacation expenses. On March 10, 1948, we traveled to New Orleans, about eighty miles distant, where we became man and wife.

We were both a young, ecstatic twenty-five and our happiness was almost complete. We also had an inner feeling of satisfaction at having circumvented a sometimes oppressive system. I somehow felt good when doing something I wasn't supposed to do.

We walked the French Quarter, looked at the city, and strolled in the park as equals with other young couples.

On our return, very little was said about our new status—in fact, nothing, to our direct knowledge. We both began to see oursevles in a new light, feeling more a part of the human race than ever before.

Our discussions became more lengthy and more in depth on the subject of eventually leaving Carville. The idea was sweet and beginning to dominate our thinking. Both of us were earning money and doing increasingly well on our tests for Hansen's disease.

So we decided to buy a grocery store in Kaplan as an investment for the future. Because of our thrifty habits, there was enough money for the purchase, and because Mom and Dad lived in Kaplan (Mom having located the investment for us), there was adequate personnel to not only mind the store, but to attend to all the other duties attendant to successfully running a business. No one was more aware than I of the strained relationship between me and the people in Kaplan, but at this point Kaplan was our projected destination when we left Carville. There was no use worrying Maria about this yet. Because of our warm and generous family support in this venture, a great deal of confidence filled our hearts.

The prospect of leaving produced mixed feelings in both of us. Carville, after all, had been our home for a great number of years. Even though life elsewhere was our fondest hope, this place had not treated us badly.

Some of the couples were permitted to build their own cottages at the back of Carville's forty-five–acre estate, and Maria and I had the opportunity to invest in a nice little place of our own. We were also able to have our meals here and dined on whatever struck our fancy.

Although happy enough in our new home, Maria, especially, became more and more obsessed with the thought of leaving. She talked about it all the time, even dreaming about it each night. I wasn't too different.

We had been married about two years when our Hansen's test results showed negative. We could leave any time we wanted. We had planned and dreamed of this day for such a long time that it was almost unbelievable. There could not be a better feeling in the whole world.

Chapter IX
Into a World That's Not Our Own

When the fateful day of departure came, I left first to find us a place to stay in Kaplan. I was filled with trepidation. The hurts and fears of my childhood had never quite left me, although, until that moment, I thought they had. I also knew that many of the rural folks I had known had moved to Kaplan in the years I was away and wondered over and over again if that boded good or ill.

We drove off and watched my little hideaway disappear behind me. Even the tall, ugly weeds growing on the riverbank looked beautiful. The whole countryside was alive with love.

The following week I bought a car. We needed transportation to bring our belongings to Kaplan from Carville. Included in our party was our dog, Rip, named in honor of my beloved hunting dog of long ago. This purchase of a car made a lot of sense, as I didn't splurge on a big luxury car or anything like that. A wise choice of a 1938 Ford was made. The engine was sound, though the body showed its age and the obvious fact that it had spent a lot of time out in all kinds of weather, as the color was impossible to determine.

The fact that I had never driven a car didn't seem to make a great deal of difference at the time. The kind salesman simply traced the gear-shifting procedures in the dust on the dashboard. Then off I went.

Nobody, living or dead, should ever accuse me of having a bad memory. I can recall in graphic and lurid detail every ache, pain, broken fingernail, unkind remark, unfair treatment, and sling and arrow of outrageous fortune that had come my way almost since my conception and—if the truth were told—could colorfully describe in detail my own birth trauma, but for some unknown reasons I didn't recall the incident of learning to ride a bike. I didn't give a thought to what Pop Smith had told me about learning safety rules and all the rest and didn't seem to remember that, when I came riding proudly back to the house at Carville, expecting praise for my new accomplishment, I had had my tail chewed out. I simply couldn't remember any of that, and with the confidence of the very young or of a raving maniac, I took off for Carville, 150 miles away, in my new car. *Wouldn't Maria be happy?* I thought (not giving a whit of recognition to the fact that she might mourn my passing if things didn't go as they should on that maiden voyage of mine as an automobile driver).

The commonplace lurches and screeches of a complaining automobile didn't bother me a bit. I just let it lurch and screech and do all those things, somehow aiming the vehicle in the general direction of Lafayette.

When I got there, in addition to the numerous other automobiles and pedestrians, I spotted a traffic light up ahead. *Damn,* I thought. *Why didn't I pay more attention before on my trips home when we came to traffic light? Was green for stop and red for go, or red for stop and green for go?* A thought crept insidiously into my mind as I poked along, shaking and anxiously looking from side to side, trying to judge what I was supposed to do by the behavior of the other drivers: "Maybe it might be a good idea to find a nice, quiet street somewhere and get a little more familiar with my Ford." I had already had some bad near-misses because I had hit the clutch when meaning to use the brake.

This new thought was comforting to me for about a millisecond. My idea had been a good one, but the surrounding traffic had absolutely no intention of allowing me to do anything except what I was already doing and neither I nor anybody else knew exactly what that was. By now I was wildly seeking a way out of this mess, reciting countless Acts of Contrition in French, English, Latin, and various admixtures thereof, facing my piety with an occasional expletive (from which, I was surprised to note, I found some comfort). A quiet street with very little traffic was finally found, and executing the most generous arc in recorded history, I managed to place myself and my car in that more serene location.

After parking the car for a few minutes, allowing my pulse to slow to about 200 pulses per minute, I decided to use this area to practice my driving skills. Never mind that I didn't know what the traffic signals meant and that I had never heard of a driver's license or insurance; I would learn to operate this infernal machine here and now.

The following several hours were spent in endless rehearsal of every maneuver imaginable. Then I tried every gear, every turn, and every kind of use of the brakes I could dream up. By the time I had found some degree of confidence, another thought found its way to my consciousness. *My God! What will I do when I have to get out on the highway with all those cars going at top speed and I don't know how to handle this automobile at speeds greater than ten miles per hour!*

I never did like making decisions, and this one was a poser. After giving the whole thing a great deal of thought, I felt I could more safely tackle the more advanced highway driving.

This noble thought was met with a small degree of success. However, I was really put out when, while I was driving on the heavily traveled Highway 90 to Baton Rouge, a frustrated motorist, finally getting a chance to pass me, stuck his head out of the window and yelled, "Get the hell off the road, old man!"

What nerve! I thought. *Calling me an old man!* A little later on, still fighting a loose front end, it occurred to me that the man had meant that I was driving like an old man.

Arriving at the cottage at four in the morning, I thought that Maria would have a stroke when she saw me. She knew, of course, that I had never driven a car, and she also knew that it took some time and practice to master the art. She was also concerned that I had been gone for God knows how long and had worried and worried.

After a while, the worry had turned to anger, working itself up to a pretty high pitch at this inconsiderate type of behavior. After the anger abated, the worry started again; then the imagination went to work; then finally the tears began flowing.

Never in her wildest dreams had she thought that her husband had bought a car and driven it many miles through all types of traffic situations and would come up to her, grinning like an idiot, expecting some kind of praise.

For all her beauty, compassion, understanding, and love, she had a mind of her own and definite ideas about things. She was also quite capable of expressing herself clearly and making sure that what she had to say was clearly understood. When she had recovered from the first shock of seeing me driving a car, she was able to put these thoughts into words that nobody, no matter how great or small the intellectual acumen, could understand.

Finally, I managed to explain that the car was for transporting our things back from Carville. Somewhat mollified, she agreed that is wasn't too bad an idea.

Men! she thought.

Women! I thought.

There seemed to be a dreamlike quality about the place. I hadn't been away all that long; still all the familiar things and people had a different feel to me—like an outgrown pair of old shoes or a bed that was too short. The well-ordered buildings and grounds, though still very attractive, now seemed artificial and unreal. Even the familiarity of our little house had an alien feel to it. I felt a push-pull about everything there.

We loaded the car pretty much in silence, neither of us quiet expressing the feeling we both shared and neither realizing at the time that we both felt the same way. The work went quickly; there was no reason to take our time.

My dearest of friends, Duffy, Carville's debonair gent, and his pretty little debutante wife, Lenore and Ellis, another oldtimer, gathered the group and gave us a going-away party.

When we had finished with that, Maria suggested that we go see some of our closer friends before the final good-bye. There were several young couples about our own age with whom we had shared good times and bad. There were also personal friends Maria and I had each had prior to our marriage and who were still close.

Maria and I found each of the people we sought, thanked them again for their farewell parties and gifts, and gave them final hugs, kisses, and handshakes, but somehow every word, every gesture, every smile seemed just out of focus. Everyone was glad to see us leave; it was just knowing that it was for the last time that put a kind of subtle strain on us all. There were a lot of long pauses where they didn't belong, and people looked at their watches when they thought nobody was looking. Everybody was happy for this young couple whose lives they had so long been a part of and shared; only now this young couple were aliens. We were no longer citizens of Carville. We were citizens of the real world, a place that the Carvillians could only vaguely remember or dream of.

I made the final visit of the day to my beloved Sister Agnes, who had been the source of so much inspiration, encouragement, and affection. Always gracious and understanding, Sister knew how to talk to me and Maria and made us feel optimistic about our future. She fussed a lot, reminding us to be sure to do this and that and not to do other things. Mainly, we were to take our medication faithfully. We both knew full well what restrictions we had on our lives, but Sister was so sweet and mother-hennish in her admonitions and her interest in us that one could only smile and feel warm toward her.

Our farewells over, Maria and I took Rip and got in the car. Not knowing if society was going to open its doors for us, in August 1950 we braved it and were off to Kaplan. The place where they lock you up and throw away the key had been challenged. Maria would mind the store, and I would find a job so we could have double income. I would not worry her about this just yet. And after giving away almost all our young adult lives to Carville, the big front steel gate had sprung open for us.

The trip, though fairly long, seemed both too short and endless. We would enthusiastically discuss plans for the future and express our love for each other. It was a new beginning for us both, and we faced it with excitement and just a twinge of dread.

When we arrived home and unpacked the car, the dream of the future was no longer a dream. This was it. The new life had now begun.

After a very short time, both Maria and I learned the ins and outs of the grocery business. When Maria had assured me that she could handle the store by herself, I set about the task of looking for a job.

In the town of Kaplan, there wasn't too much in the way of work I could do. Even though I was free of Hansen's disease, there were many taboos remaining that made things difficult for me. Perseverance was important, and I took very little time during the day practicing anything else.

From time to time, I would drive to the site of my former home. Nothing was the same anymore. The road leading to the house had been plowed under, and brush had grown where the house once was. The old well was standing above the weeds. How many times as a child had I grabbed the tip of that handle and pumped water to wash my feet?

It was apparent that I would have to move on to a larger city to find employment. So I decided to try Lake Charles, which had a reputation for being in need of a lot of help. I went there eagerly seeking a position that I could fill. The only problem was that it was impossible to explain that I had spent my life in Carville since the age of fifteen, because I feared the information would preclude any possibility of employment, even if I said I had been discharged.

Therefore I found it necessary to invent previous situations held and to give ficticious references on job interviews. I had no idea whether there was any kind of follow-up on this or not.

On May 1, 1951, I was hired on the spot when I applied for work in a supermarket. My few months of self-employed grocery experience helped me qualify for the job. The work varied and I was soon doing a commendable job.

Since it was too far to commute, I found a small apartment so that Maria could be with me. She could find a job here, and we could continue the pursuit of our goals.

Maria soon joined me, and things went very nicely for us both. My work was more than satisfactory, and in no time my efforts were rewarded with a promotion. Mom was tending the store, life was going along splendidly, and Maria and I were happy and optimistic.

On my way to work one day, I stopped at a filling station to fill up. Then I discovered that the owner of the station was a former grounds-keeper at Carville whom I knew well. When the mutual discovery was made, there were handshakes and a lot of "Isn't it a small world?" We chatted warmly, as old friends would want to do, and with a smile on my face and a song on my lips, I proceeded on to work.

Five days after this meeting with my friend, Mr. Sudden, I was called to the boss's office and summarily dismissed: "D. J., you cannot work for us any more." No reason was given and no matter how insistently I questioned the boss, no answer was forthcoming, only evasions.

I was so devastated at this sudden unexpected turn of events, that I forgot myself and my dignity and pleaded with the boss to reconsider and said that whatever I did wrong would be amended. It was to no avail.

In a state of complete despair and confusion, all I could think about was how badly life had treated me. I virtually wallowed in self-pity and contemplated the paucity of compassion and understanding I was receiving from the man who previously had been so complimentary and encouraging to me. Inwardly, I railed at how unfair everything was.

After a protracted period of this pathological behavior and thinking, I realized that Maria would have to be told about this persecution. With a heavy heart, I proceeded homeward.

When Maria came to the door to greet me with her customary kiss, she was taken aback by my disoriented behavior and somnolent appearance.

I began sobbing and trembling and was inconsolable. It was only with the greatest of tact and understanding that Maria was able to elicit the reason for my feeling so low.

Upon her learning the facts, we both cried in each other's arms. Maria, as usual, showed great strength and warmly reassured and reminded me of God's own love and compassion as well as her own. Her faith was constant and above reproach. She knew the right things to say and do. I was again able to remind myself of how very fortunate I was to have the love of this wonderful woman.

After a long conversation, during which much support and encouragement was given to me, we decided to try another place where Carville and all its unvenerated connotations, we hoped, would not be known. We chose a larger city, four hundred miles away, San Antonio, Texas. Maybe we would change our names and not give anyone our address and phone number.

The next day, we were off to our new home. We felt like two criminals at large, running and hiding to stay alive, but vivacious and exuberant with this extra security. We talked about and felt fortunate that Mr. Sudden had chosen not to report me to Carville and have me brought back there again.

We had, as a chilling reminder, previously witnessed handcuffed patients being brought back at gunpoint by the law.

The trip was long and hot, and so was San Antonio this July 4, 1951. We found an apartment fairly quickly and settled down in it and immediately began job hunting.

Within a very short time, we each found work—I in a supermarket and Maria as a bookkeeper in a shoe factory. Of course our references were falsified, and though my new position paid slightly less than the previous one, our combined salaries (sixty-five dollars per week) gave us security in our new beginning.

Now, a little more nervous about people knowing me, I started to work with great enthusiasm and vigor, and again my employers were taken with my conscious efforts and enthusiasm for my job. Maria, too, was greatly appreciated in her position. Both of us eagerly applied ourselves, no detail being overlooked in our efforts to constantly improve our work.

As the months passed, we made new and satisfying friendships, both at work and in our neighborhood and at church. We were to do many things we had never done before and were very happy and content.

As our sense of security deepened, Maria and I started discussing our cherished dream of owning our own home, although having our names registered at the courthouse wasn't appealing. We had both seen places that we liked, and when the discussion became really serious, we began to actively look for a house to buy.

The place we wanted was easy enough to find and so was the realtor who wanted to sell it to us. We were delighted with our prospective home and ready to move in until the down payment was mentioned. Once again disappointment raised its ugly head, and a cloak of despair fell about our shoulders. I felt so helpless and worried that Maria would be more disappointed than me. We hadn't known what a down payment was, but had just wanted to pay sixty-five dollars monthly and move in.

In her characteristic and understanding but practical way, Maria came to the rescue in yet another unhappy situation. She told me that she felt that we had been so blessed since moving to San Antonio and even before, when our tests for Hansen's had proven negative, that a short wait until the accumulated amount of money necessary for the down payment was obtained would be worthwhile. She pointed out that it would be yet another goal for us and reminded me of the sense of exhilaration we both felt each time even the smallest of victories was accomplished.

Now there was yet another project to tackle, and we both worked to that end, saving each penny we could. After what seemed like forever, the money was saved, and in 1952 Maria and I moved onto our very own home. We couldn't have been happier. Now we could make this place into exactly the home we had wished for and dreamed of for such a long time.

The lawn was done to perfection, as were the shrubbery and the roses and other flowers, artistically arranged in tasteful profusion. The years at Carville, when I saw how the nuns cared for the flowers there, paid off. Maria had decorated the inside of the house with beautiful colors, putting up exquisite drapes, which she had sewn herself. As both of us were very artistic, our decorating made manifest our talents. Maria, with her impeccable taste in colors and interior decorating, and I, with my keen eye for nature, made the home a showplace. We, a happy couple, felt that our lives were just about complete and we had about everything anyone could ever want.

After a little over a year in our new home, I experienced some pain in my left arm. Of course I was immediately concerned that HD was back knocking on my door again. I couldn't abide the thought of the disease or of having to return to the hospital now that my life was in order and things were going so well for me. There was so much we would lose if I had to quit work. The house, the furniture, and even the clothes on our back were not paid off. Perhaps, I thought the pain would go away. I even reasoned that the pain might be due to some strain sustained at work or when doing the yard, so decided to pay no attention to it for the time being.

The pain, however, remained and began to intensify, and the only course of action now was to go to Carville and have it checked.

On my arrival there, the doctor looked me over and comfirmed that I did indeed have a recurrence of HD, but it was not necessary for me to remain there. Years of technological research at Carville had revealed that the disease was mildly transmittable, if at all. He said I could return home and continue to work and live much the same way I had, but *must* take prescribed medication and get more rest. Then I was given a larger dose of a derivative of the medication I had been taking when I left Carville, called Diasone, along with sedatives and painkillers. My instructions were to return every six months to be checked. That wasn't really so bad, and, as my worse fears had been confirmed and allayed at the same time, my return to San Antonio was a very optimistic one.

Life went on for me and Maria much as it had been going on, with the exception of my twice-yearly visits to Carville. It turned out that I was resistant to the medication I was receiving, and other forms of medication were tried. I was still able to work, so in spite of a good many more symptoms making themselves known, I continued to do so.

After several years, Maria and I realized that our beautiful home, which we both loved so dearly and on which we had lavished so much care, wasn't big enough anymore. Aside from our own accumulation of furnituure, we had many out-of-town guests and no place to put them, so the decision to buy a larger home was reluctantly made. My physical condition, by now, was improving, and I was working steadily. When we located the spacious home we wanted, we rented out the one-bedroom house we were living in and bought and moved into the new one, in 1956.

If this LeBeaux family had been enthusiastic in moving into their first home, it was nothing compared to the zeal with which they attacked the one they now occupied. Not a detail was overlooked or ignored. Meticulous as always, Maria found details where none existed and saw to it that they were attended to. She was adamant on the subject of coordinating colors, and all had to be exact. She was equally perspicacious in her housekeeping duties. If ever a perfect wife existed, it was Maria, and above all, people knew it. With her, the simplest pleasures were cherished. To be with Maria was to be in the company of an angel, and when she spoke, everything seemed to become right. Her gentle, pious ways, her steadfast devotions, and her love and loyalty to me, her husband, put her in a class by herself. Add to this her sensual beauty and natural charm and grace and no one could ever wonder why I found her to be the most wonderful person ever. She never had made an effort to acquire these traits that made her enchanting. She was, in fact, quite unaware of them, wanting only to lead the life of a good Catholic and good wife. That natural intelligence of hers served her well and came to her rescue on the many occasions that my illnesses threatened our perfect marriage.

I was working diligently, hoping to get the position of assistant manager at the store where I was employed. My efforts were rewarded when I was promoted to assistant manager in 1957. With careful investments in real estate, Maria and I were able to realize a nice profit. The financial picture for us was very good, and now when we worried, for the first time it wasn't because of limited means.

Each visit made to Carville showed improvement in my health. We also saw new and better things for the patients there. Because the disease was not considered communicable, as it once was, there were fewer and fewer restrictions placed upon the patients and most of them came and went at will. They also were free to marry. Some married doctors, nurses, other patients, and so on and owned their own cars to travel to town. In Carville's sixty-year history, only one employee has contracted the malady, and doubts are still overshadowing the authenticity of a correct diagnosis. Simple precautions are taken, as at any other hospitals. There are two things that are not affected by this disease: the sex drive and the mind. About five thousand intellectually stable patients are living in society many with children of their own.

Many scientics believe that HD is hereditary and a person must have a special vulnerability to the particular bacilli in order to develop it. Skin discolorations, areas of insensitivity, sunstrokes, ringworm, mild joint pains, feeling feverish, et cetera could all be signs, and the victim should be directed to appropriate channels for treatments.

The people who lived at Carville permanently were mainly those whose handicaps were too advanced before help came along and who had no other place they could survive.

Health improving and income better, I started thinking of ways in which I could do better financially and not have to spend so many hours working . After many considerations, I took a few correspondence courses in IBM training, then finally went into computers. I worked all day at the supermarket and did my lessons at night. It was a grueling schedule, but it paid off and in 1959 I received my diploma in the science of computer programming.

The following year I went to work for the U.S. Air force. The civil-service physical had me rather worried, but the worry proved unnecessary, as I passed with flying colors.

When I first began working, it was on the "graveyard" shift (12:00 P.M.– 8:00 A.M.). The new hours began to take their toll, and my old nemesis started creeping back. Ready to panic or cut and run, I was almost at loggerheads with the situation. Then I had the chance to go to work in Supply during the usual working hours and took it. This helped enormously. During the next four years, twelve more courses related to my job were completed. Never far from my thinking was the possibility of promotion should my efforts be recognized. All of this was not without its setbacks, however. Hansen's disease had hit me with a vengeance. I was in pain most of the time and running a high fever. I was also beginning to show outward physical symptoms that were hard not to notice. That unstylish LeBeauxdachi look was coming back. My hands would swell, making it almost impossible to operate the delicate equipment I used. My face didn't look so good, either, I carried a large supply of pills with me, which I had to use just to get through the day sometimes.

My trips to Carville indicated that I was more or less immune to the medications I was using, and others had to be substituted.

In the meantime, taking sick leave was almost impossible, so much of it had been taken when I was running a fever or having pains, so I just had to tough it out. I was fully aware that the researchers at Carville were working long hours developing new technology for the treatment and containment of my disease, and the thought of that was sometimes the only thing that kept me going. Actually, it was that and my own awareness of my drug dependency, which, necessary or not, was very real.

Maria, in the meantime, was doing more than ever before. In addition to all her responsibilities with home and career, she now was also nursing her increasingly dependent husband through night after night of physical and mental suffering. Had I at any time accepted my situation for what it was, I might have spared myself and my devoted wife a lot, but I hadn't, and after all these years, was forcing myself and my wife to endure hardships that would have to be experienced to be appreciated.

On my next visit to Carville, I got the unpleasant news that I had developed a nonreversible renal disease in addition to HD. There was no way to avoid the consequences, and I was given a life expectancy of three to four years at best.

The medics advised me to get my affairs in order, pay all bills and insurance premiums, and make my peace with God. I was also reminded to make my will forthwith. My condition (amyloid) was similar to leukemia in its effects. Maria and I grasped the point, which was impossible to miss.

On our return trip, most of our communication was nonverbal. I was sure of how Maria must have felt. She didn't have much to say and kept her own counsel. I knew, of course, that she must have been suffering, much as my mother had suffered from the time she had learned of my condition until the day she died.

We made a stop in Lafayette to see our old friends, Father Louis and his faithful housekeeper, Elvira. Father Louis had known both me and Maria during our brief stay in Kaplan when he was stationed there and had commiserated with our dilemma. This night, he gave us comfort in his own particular way. Father Louis had a way of making one interested in any subject. Whilst doing this little exercise, he would usually manage not only to raise the spirits, but to bring a smile to the lips and, by the end of his (sometimes pedantic) dialogue, provoke the old Cajun knee-slapping laughter in the most inconsolable of his supplicants.

In spite of my gallant efforts to let nothing take my mind off my own tragic predicament, I found myself responding, reluctantly, to Father Louis's methods.

He was an ingenious man and took an intellectual approach to all things, including spiritual matters.

It was not surprising that when Father Louis lapsed into prose or poetry, he was not always understood. He would, more or less, quote Longfellow when he said, more or less, "Life is great! Life is earnest! and the grave is not its goal."

After returning to San Antonio, I took care of the mundane tasks the doctors had recommended, i.e., got my affairs in order, paid insurance premiums, made a will. I accomplished these things with an inspired lack of enthusiasm, my thoughts being constantly on my own problems and how unfairly life had always treated me.

I flailed about, trying to find ways to escape my own tortured thoughts, and my self-pity was as much a part of me as my fingernails. I visited relatives and tried a few leisurely pastimes, such as fishing or hunting, but these activities only gave me more time for more introspection, my thoughts feeding on themselves like a snake swallowing its tail.

Then I found a few answers, looking in the bottom of a whiskey bottle. Before long, my nodding acquaintance with the old Four Roses had become a fast friendship. It made me feel better, and enough of it made the suffering go away. My liquor bottle and I spent the days together. All possible precautions were taken to keep my guilty secret from Maria, and I was convinced that I was successful in my attempts. There were all manners of caches where my supply seemed innocuous enough, and I had elaborate schemes for the disposal of all the "dead soldiers." The bottles were pulverized and mixed with sawdust.

I was so clever and devised intricate dodges to cloak my true actions. Sometimes I would go to the workshop and turn on all the electrical equipment to show Maria that I was slaving away at some complicated project. In the meantime, I would be laid back, getting myself back to "normal."

This unholy alliance went on unchecked for years. I greeted my friendly bottle the first thing when I came home from work evenings and the last thing before I went to bed. There were never any occasions when the two of us weren't together, even at work.

One day the good old Duffys from Carville came to visit us. It was an unexpected, but welcome visit. Our conversation, quite naturally, turned to the subject of Hansen's disease and the current treatments. My ears perked up when our friends told us about a new medication that was being tried and had had 100 percent effective cures.

On learning this piece of information, I lost no time in going to Carville and volunteering for the new treatment. The drug turned out to be all that had been said of it. How great a contribution the Duffys made to my life they will never know.

I also stopped drinking, cold turkey, at this point. The withdrawal symptoms were undescribably painful, but I didn't have the alcohol in my bloodstream all the time, complicating the effects of the medicines I was taking. Sufficient motivation was mustered to attain these more important goals. Besides, I couldn't have handled my life without extraordinary aches, pains, and suffering, but that hurdle was soon passed and, in an unusually short time, the awful symptoms abated and I was once again on the road to recovery. This heroic reversal took place in the Year of Our Lord 1967.

With improving health, I once more set my sights on improving my personal and economic situation. The only physical problem I now had was a troublesome stomach. When that problem remained with me for an unreasonable length of time, I consulted a local physician, who referred me to a psychiatrist. The psychiatrist, after lengthy consultation, determined that I was suffering from a severe mental disorder brought about by my troubled past. My rejections, family deprivation as a youth, and the countless lows and highs of my past had made my mind sick. This sick mind was making my nerves sick. My sick nerves were making my stomach sick. The sick stomach would lower the person's appetite and create, in general, a weakening, uncoordinated condition. So I was given shock treatments.

Once a week for two months, I drove to the hospital to take the treatments. My condition was stress-related, as I could easily believe.

A month after the conclusion of the shock treatments, I had to go to Carville for my routine checkup. I was told by the new and competent Dr. La Pearl that my stomach trouble had been caused not by emotional problems, but by the kidney condition itself.

The number of years had long passed since the original allotted time for renal failure, and privately, I thought that that diagnosis, too, had been in error. Again, my life continued to improve. My stomach settled, and my thoughts turned to my most cherished hope. More than anything else, I wanted a college degree. After meticulous planning to achieve that end, I again went back to Carville to make sure that my health would not interfere with my new plans. Fortunately, the results checked out almost perfectly.

I now had only one fear, and that was that as I had not graduated from high school, I would not be accepted in a university. I remembered that Elvira had told us about a fire in a small town nearby that had destroyed the local high school, burning it to the ground with all the records.

Armed with this information, I enrolled in college, citing my graduation from the now nonexistent high school in Louisiana. The year I used was 1940, because that was when I would have graduated had it not been for Hansen's disease. This seemed to work, and I was accepted as a student.

I passed the physical with no trouble. The entrance exam was another matter, however. Even though I did poorly on that, I was allowed to remain a student and I began my life as a college man at the age of fifty-three.

No academic records were set, so far as grades were concerned, but I did manage to hang in there and buck the odds. It wasn't easy, of course. Aside from the obvious problem of over forty years' absence from a classroom, I worked full time, so my time had to be quite well organized. It was necessary to use each moment to its fullest and not waste a second.

Maria, of course, gave me her full support and cooperation. She even enrolled in some courses herself, studying law enforcement, and she and I attended some of her classes together, though my major was psychology. My grades continued to improve, and we were both very pleased with the way things were going.

After I had completed two years of college, it was time for another trip to Carville. Dr. La Pearl by this time was very familiar with my case and had done a lot of research and study on the kidney problem I had. Though I felt quite well and had had little or no symptoms of the kidney condition, the test results proved otherwise. I was told to find a good kidney specialist in San Antonio and give him all details of my health background and current tests' findings. I was to be prepared to go on dialysis in the very near future.

Needless to say, I reacted badly to the news, but I was determined to continue my education and try to attain the goals I had set out for myself.

Upon returning to San Antonio, I took a week off from work and school and Maria and I took a long-awaited vacation to Florida. We'd find romance and moments of enchantment, Maria and I, by having a sandwich in a roadside park. We had had to do with so little all our lives that a sandwich, a soda, and a bonding togetherness made the whole experience rich and complete.

Things continued to go well for close to a year. It was then that I became quite ill one night and had to be rushed to the hospital. The problem was with a kidney stone—unrelated to the kidney condition, acutally—but it was decided that since I was in the hospital and since the renal disorder was so advanced, now was the time to implant a fistula in my arm so dialysis treatments could begin.

The dialysis was three times a week, four hours each time. My general health improved with each treatment, with the help of other medications administered, and I used the time when connected to the machine to do my studies and paperwork. After treatments, I was off to work, then to classes. I made my traditional stop at a little Spanish restaurant in an atmosphere of Spanish-style decoration, including the famous yellow candlelight gaily dancing around the walls while the music played.

After a year of hemodialysis, a new treatment (peritoneal dialysis) was tried, with an artificial kidney around the waist. But as in most cases, my body rejected the implanted tubings used for the treatment and a raging infection ensued. I missed a lot of school because of this, but after the tubes were surgically removed and I went back to hemodialysis, I was again able to return to classes and continue with my job and education.

Finally, in May 1979, I got my bachelor's degree in psychology, only five years after I had started school. I was ecstatic. The impossible feat was no more. A man with a fifth-grade education had entered and completed college.

Filled with enthusiasm at having completed my undergraduate studies, I decided to continue in graduate school and try for a master's in industrial psychology. Glowing with optimism, I enrolled that fall. Graduate school proved to be quite different from college, however. By the end of the first semester, I realized that there was no way I could handle the course requirements, so I had to withdraw as a student.

It was also at that time that I resigned from the air force. The continued schedule of work, study, and dialysis was too much for me, and at this point, this resignation did not signal the same kind of running away I had done on other occasions. It made sense, for a change, as I was really frail at this point.

With more time and fewer responsibilities, I hoped to regain some strength. I was given the assurance that I could do just that if I had a kidney transplant.

Dr. La Pearl asked me to ask May, my sister, to give me one of her kidneys, because a relative donor is usually more compatible. May replied with a big "YES" after consulting with her husband. She was fully aware of all the possible problems that would arise from the transplant, but, with the support of her husband, insisted. As it turned out, after lengthy testing, she was a perfect match.

When I met with the chief transplant surgeon in San Antonio, my request was turned down. Even after reassurances were obtained from Dr. La Pearl at Carville that HD would not flare up with rejection medications, I was still denied surgery. In desperation. I called Carville and was told by Dr. Jacobson, director of medicine, to find another doctor. "If Dr. Alexander does not want to give you a transplant, we cannot make him," he said.

I found a new doctor in Houston. It was necessary to make many trips there, two hundred miles away and for my sisters and

I to undergo countless tests. There was still another delay when they decided to remove my spleen to forestall the possibility of rejecting the new kidney and the convalescence from that surgery, but finally those obstacles were out of the way and the day arrived for transplantation.

Not only was the surgery a great success, but I now have the distinction of being the first and only American with Hansen's disease to undergo such surgery. Two more operations were successfully completed in Europe. After the incredibly brief stay at the hospital, I returned to San Antonio, feeling better than I had in my whole life and looking better, too. Having a new kidney and knowing that I was just a hair away from complete recovery for HD, I was genuinely happy. I was warned about the symptoms of organ rejections but, feeling the way I did, didn't worry.

After being home for a week, I was overtaken by the first rejection. Houston was notified and I was told to get there at once. Reacting with my usual panic, I called Maria at work to tell her. She rushed home, threw a few articles of clothing in a suitcase, and took off immediately for the Hermann Hospital in Houston. Then I was given antirejection medicines, radiation therapy, and numerous other treatments in the hospital. Maria could only stay there three days and had to return home after that time. In the meantime, I cooperated completely and my condition improved dramatically. In two weeks' time she came to Houston and brought me home.

Then I was home for less than a day when the trip to the hospital was repeated. This time I had spots on my lungs (a fungus) and had to stay for over eight weeks before the condition was cleared up. In short, I had to return to Houston a total of seven times during that year because of possible rejection of the new kidney, et cetera. Sixteen operations later, it was no use wishing and hoping anymore. In June of 1982, a year to the day after the initial transplant, the new kidney failed completely. All the efforts by the medics to revive the kidney did not work.

Now I had to go back on dialysis again.

Actually, the regularity of the three days a week was at least predictable, whereas the trips back and forth to Houston were not. I received offers of kidneys, from every family member, but declined them, opting, instead, to be placed on the list for cadaver donors. Just to be sure, my name was entered on the list in Houston, New Orleans, and San Antonio, and as of now, I am still waiting to hear from either source. Dr. Alexander, the San Antonio surgeon, reconsidered and now agreed to go through with the operation whenever a donor would be available.

I never saw Gleanda again, but she always will have a special place in my heart, as only a first love can have. I am well aware that the love that Maria and I share is real and strong, but sometimes my thoughts drift back to that small schoolhouse and that sweet little girl sitting in front of me.

Mom died of cancer in 1960.

My father and Darbee developed Hansen's disease and went to Carville for treatments. Both became immune to the available drugs and died before the new 100 percent effective drug, B663, was in use. They both suffered kidney failure. I am still taking the drug and doing fine.

Uncle Yas bought the farmhouse and the grocery store in Kaplan. He is now dead.

Most aunts and uncles have passed on, and with the exception of Darbee, the rest of the LeBeaux children, including our adopted sister Teresa, and a boy Tom, who lived with us, are alive and well.

I now spend my time, when not in dialysis, in a great effort trying to educate and inform people about Hansen's disease. I realize now that many of the things that made me so miserable were of my own invention. I just didn't give people a chance to be my friends, but gave too much of myself toward living in the past. The fact that I developed a peculiar outlook on life is unimportant. The fact that I now know it and want more than anything else to try and prevent it happening to someone else is what matters.

Maria has never lost her spirit or her faith. Though she saw me through the worst possible of times, she has remained relatively untouched by life's indignities. We now share, in addition to our all-consuming love and devotion to one another, an unyielding faith in God and the future.

Thank you for walking with me. It has been a long journey. If we ever meet again, come over and say hello. I would like that.

NOTE: Outpatients' Hansen's disease clinics in the Continental United States are strategically located in Los Angeles, San Francisco, San Diego, Seattle, New York, Boston, Carville, New Orleans, Miami, and Chicago. New HD sulphone drugs available include Dapsone, Rifampin, B663, Ethionamide, Thalidomide, Corticosteriod, Transfer Factor, and others.